The Pen, The Stethoscope, and The Scalpel

Ogochukwu M. Cox

The Pen, The Stethoscope, and The Scalpel

Women Physician Writers and Their Profound Impact on Medicine and Society

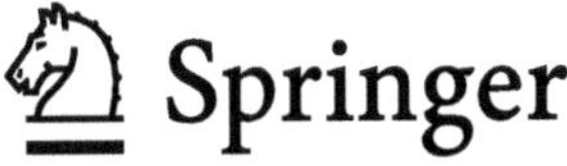
Springer

Ogochukwu M. Cox
Pediatric Cardiology
University of Massachusetts
Worcester, MA, USA

ISBN 978-3-032-19405-3 ISBN 978-3-032-19406-0 (eBook)
https://doi.org/10.1007/978-3-032-19406-0

This Springer imprint is published by the registered company Springer Nature Switzerland AG
The registered company address is: Gewerbestrasse 11, 6330 Cham, Switzerland

Contents

Chapter 1
Elisabeth Kübler-Ross, MD

Following much internal debate over which iconic physician-author should open this list of female masters of Arts and Science, I recalled a question once posed to my residency class by a visiting professor. "What is the difference between a physician and a patient?" The answer? Time. I have had the dubious privilege, myself, of being admitted to the ICU, and the humbling honor of having chronic medical conditions requiring lifelong communication with specialist physicians. This is along with necessary knowledge acquisition of the medical insurance industry and grueling practice navigating the intricacies of state-by-state rules regarding pharmacies versus Durable Medical Equipment companies. I was one of the first people to murmur the word "time," into our conference room that midday, in the brief period before the professor advanced the slide deck to the four-letter-word. Time.

When I think about time, I think about Dr. Elisabeth Kübler-Ross, who famously described the stages of grief. Denial and isolation, anger, bargaining, depression, and acceptance. I learned about Dr. Kübler-Ross in a psychology class while at university and then reflected on those stages shortly after, when my grandmother passed away. I have since learned more about the doctor, and it would be my honor to share that knowledge with you.

Dr. Elisabeth Kübler-Ross was born in Zurich, Switzerland on July 8th, 1926, to Ernst and Emma Villiger Kübler, and moved to the United States in 1958 [1]. She entered the world as part of a set of triplets, three daughters born to a middle-class Swiss family on a summer day in 1926 [1, 2]. Her arrival was, at the time, by medical accounts, precarious. Weighing two pounds at birth, she and one of her sisters hovered between life and death in those critical first hours and days [2, 3]. That she survived at all, Kübler-Ross would later credit to her mother's close attention and love [1, 3]. Her early life would come to involve other brushes with mortality, which may have established death, in her view, as one of the necessary experiences of being on this earth. Her early childhood encounters with the concept of death, may also have foreshadowed her eventual dedication to a career in understanding the end of life.

O. M. Cox, *The Pen, The Stethoscope, and The Scalpel*,
https://doi.org/10.1007/978-3-032-19406-0_1

Growing up as a triplet proved to be both a blessing and a burden. The three girls became minor celebrities in Zurich, their faces appearing in advertisements throughout the city [3, 4]. Yet this public attention came at a cost that young Elisabeth felt keenly. She was rarely called by her own name, instead being lumped together with her sisters as simply "the Kübler triplets [3, 5]." This lack of individual recognition affected her profoundly, sparking what she later described as an independent, rebellious streak. The experience of being seen but not truly recognized as an individual would inform her later work, where she insisted on treating each dying patient as a unique person with their own story, not merely as a case of terminal illness [4].

The Kübler household was dominated by their father, whose firmness was balanced by tenderness with his daughters; singing songs around the parlor piano and leading them on summer nature hikes at the family's mountain retreat in Furlegi [3, 4]. These excursions instilled in young Elisabeth, a lasting love and respect for nature that she carried throughout her life [4]. She found solace atop a flat rock in the woods near her home, a secret place where she could escape the constant company of her sisters and simply be herself [3, 4]. Even as an adult, she would return to this spot when in need of peace and reflection.

By the sixth grade, Elisabeth had decided she wanted to become a doctor. This aspiration met fierce resistance from her father, who believed medicine was not the pursuit for a girl. He insisted she should either become a secretary in his office supply business or pursue the traditional path of housekeeping [3, 4]. The confrontation between father and daughter represented a clash between old world expectations and a young woman's determination to forge her own path. At 16 years old, Elisabeth made the bold decision that would define her character: she left home [3, 6].

What followed were years that would shape not only her practical skills but her fundamental understanding of human suffering. Elisabeth supported herself through various jobs; as a cook, a mason, a roofer, and an assistant at an eye clinic [1]. During World War II, at just 13, she worked as a laboratory assistant for refugees in Zurich [3, 6]. These experiences brought her face to face with the displaced, and the dying. She witnessed firsthand how war stripped away everything people held dear, yet also how the human spirit could endure unimaginable hardship.

When the war ended in 1945, 19-year-old Elisabeth joined the International Voluntary Service for Peace as an activist [3]. She traveled across Eastern Europe, helping to rebuild devastated communities and set up first-aid clinics in war-torn countries [1]. She met refugees and survivors of concentration camps, listening to their stories of loss and survival. One visit in particular, appeared to change her forever: the Majdanek concentration camp in Poland, where more than 300,000 people had died. Walking through that place of unspeakable horror, Elisabeth saw drawings on the walls: butterflies sketched by children who knew they were going to die [1]. These butterflies would become a recurring symbol in her later work, representing transformation and the fragile beauty of life in the face of death.

The experience at Majdanek seemingly crystallized something in Elisabeth. She would spend her life healing others, bringing dignity and compassion to those who suffered. In 1951, against her father's wishes but with unshakable determination, she enrolled in the medical school at the University of Zurich [1, 3].

Medical school brought more than just education; it brought love. Elisabeth met Emanuel Robert Ross, an American medical student, and found in him a kindred spirit [1]. They married in 1958, shortly after she graduated with her medical degree [1, 3]. The newlyweds moved to New York, where both began internships at Glen Cove Community Hospital on Long Island [1, 3]. For Elisabeth, it meant leaving behind her beloved Switzerland, the mountains she had hiked as a child, and that flat rock where she had found solace. But America represented opportunity, a chance to practice medicine in new ways and on a larger scale.

Elisabeth began her psychiatric residency at Manhattan State Hospital on July 6, 1959, marking the beginning of a career that would revolutionize how medicine approached death [1, 3]. What she found in American hospitals disturbed her deeply. Patients who were dying were treated with what she saw as shocking neglect and lack of compassion. They were isolated, ignored, and left alone with their fear and pain. Doctors would not even provide adequate pain medication, worried about the possibility of addiction in patients who had only weeks or months to live [3]. The medical community, so focused on saving lives, seemed utterly unable or unwilling to deal with those who were dying.

This approach stood in stark contrast to what Elisabeth had known in Switzerland, where death was considered a natural part of the life cycle and people typically died at home, surrounded by family and friends [7]. She was appalled by what she called the "layer of professional denial [8]" that prohibited patients from expressing their innermost concerns. Medical schools, she discovered, taught "everything about your liver and nothing about you as a person [9]."

In 1962, Elisabeth and her husband moved to Denver, where she accepted a teaching position at the University of Colorado School of Medicine. That same year, she became an American citizen [6]. It was in Denver that she began to truly find her voice as an advocate for the dying. When asked to fill in for a colleague one day, she made what would prove to be a revolutionary decision: she brought a 16-year-old girl, dying from leukemia, into the classroom and interviewed her in front of the medical students [1, 6].

The interview was raw, honest, and moving. The young girl spoke openly about her fears, anger, sadness, and hopes. She was not presented as a case study or an example of pathology, but as a human being trying to make sense of what was happening to her. Elisabeth's intention was to show her students that dying patients were not just bodies with failing organs, but people with thoughts, feelings, and a profound need to be heard and understood. As she told her students that day: "Now you are reacting like human beings instead of scientists. Maybe now you'll not only know how a dying patient feels, but you will also be able to treat them with compassion. The same compassion that you would want for yourself [10]."

The response was powerful. Students began to see dying patients differently, and word of Elisabeth's innovative teaching method spread. By 1966, her Death and Dying seminars were gaining larger audiences and earning her academic popularity. The Lutheran Theological Seminary invited her to join their staff as a counselor in pastoral care, recognizing that future pastors needed training in how to minister effectively to the terminally ill and dying [1].

In 1965, the Kübler-Ross family moved to Chicago, where Elisabeth became an assistant professor of psychiatry at Billings Hospital, affiliated with the University of Chicago [3]. She continued her groundbreaking work, holding a series of well-attended seminars in which terminally ill patients were interviewed and allowed to express themselves freely [3, 7]. She listened to them with a depth of attention that was rare in medicine at the time. She asked them about their fears, their regrets, their unfinished business, and their hopes. And in their answers, she began to see patterns emerging.

Years of research, hundreds of hours spent at the bedsides of dying patients, countless conversations—all of this culminated in Elisabeth Kübler-Ross's landmark book, "On Death and Dying," published in 1969 [11]. In it, she described what she had observed through her work: five psychological stages that terminally ill patients commonly experienced as they processed their diagnosis and approached death.

The stages were:

Denial "It can't be happening to me." This initial stage served as a temporary defense mechanism, a buffer against the overwhelming reality of a terminal diagnosis [11].

Anger "Why me? How dare you do this to me?" Patients directed their rage at God, at themselves, at their doctors, at anyone they perceived as responsible for their suffering [11].

Bargaining "Just let me live to see my daughter's wedding." Patients attempted to negotiate with fate, with God, with the universe, seeking to postpone the inevitable [11].

Depression "I'm so sad. Why bother with anything?" As the reality set in, patients grappled with deep sadness and a sense of hopelessness [11].

Acceptance "I know that I will be in a better place." Finally, many patients reached a place of peace with their fate, ready to face what came next with dignity [11].

Dr. Kübler-Ross was careful to note in her work that not all patients experienced all five stages, nor did they necessarily experience them in this order. Some patients might move between stages or remain in one stage for an extended period [11]. The framework was meant to be a lens, a tool to help caregivers understand and respond to what their patients were going through, not a rigid prescription for how people "should" grieve.

The book became an instant bestseller, resonating far beyond the medical community [3, 6]. In November 1969, Life magazine published an article about Kübler-Ross and her work, bringing public awareness to her revolutionary approach [1, 3]. The response was overwhelming [4]. Here was someone willing to break the taboo, to talk openly about death in a culture that had sanitized and hidden it away. Suddenly, death was no longer unmentionable. People began to discuss it in living rooms, in churches, and in classrooms. And Elisabeth Kübler-Ross became a household name.

The impact on medicine was profound and lasting. By July 1982, Kübler-Ross had taught 125,000 students in death and dying courses at colleges, seminaries, medical schools, hospitals, and social work institutions across the country and around the world [3, 4]. Her work inspired a new field of study called thanatology: the study of death and dying [4]. Medical schools began including courses on death and dying in their curricula. Psychologists, sociologists, anthropologists, and theologians all began researching death-related behavior with new vigor and perspective.

Perhaps most significantly, Kübler-Ross became a champion of the worldwide hospice movement. Throughout the 1970s, she traveled to over 20 countries on 6 continents, initiating various hospice and palliative care programs [1, 3]. She was instrumental in helping to establish more than 50 hospices globally [8]. These facilities represented a radical departure from traditional hospital care, focusing not on cure but on comfort, not on extending life at all costs but on ensuring quality of life in whatever time remained.

In 1970, she delivered the prestigious Ingersoll Lecture on Human Immortality at Harvard University, bringing academic gravitas to the subject of death and dying [3, 4]. Two years later, on August 7, 1972, she spoke to the United States Senate Special Committee on Aging, promoting the "Death With Dignity" movement [3]. Her testimony helped influence public policy regarding end–of–life care, palliative medicine, and patients' rights [1].

Dr. Kübler-Ross's influence extended into the emerging field of clinical ethics in ways that are still felt today [12]. She fundamentally changed the context, content, and process of clinical ethics by placing the patient's experience and voice—not merely the patient's pathology—at the center of medical concern [12]. She taught caregivers to pay attention to the importance of process and interpersonal communication in patient care. In doing so, she prepared the soil in which the discipline of clinical ethics took root and grew well beyond her original focus [12].

Her work also had practical implications for how doctors communicated with patients. Before Dr. Kübler-Ross, it was common practice to withhold terminal diagnoses from patients, operating under the paternalistic belief that such knowledge would be harmful [4]. Dr. Kübler-Ross argued passionately that patients had the right to know their prognosis and that honest communication, delivered with compassion, allowed patients to make peace with their situation, finish unfinished business, and die with dignity [11].

Always thinking of the most overlooked and vulnerable, Dr. Kübler-Ross expanded her advocacy in unexpected directions. In the mid-1980s, she initiated the concept of prison hospice, beginning work with incarcerated populations in Vacaville, California, and later in prisons in Ireland and Scotland [1]. Her work in these facilities laid the foundation for a major shift in how dying inmates are treated, emphasizing their right to dignity and humane care even while incarcerated.

During the early days of the AIDS epidemic, when fear and stigma surrounded the disease, Kübler-Ross worked tirelessly with AIDS patients [1]. She attempted to create a hospice specifically for AIDS-afflicted children but encountered fierce opposition from communities unwilling to have such a facility in their neighborhoods. The rejection hurt her deeply, but it did not stop her advocacy [10].

In 1977, funded by profits from her books, workshops, and speaking engagements, she established Shanti Nilaya (Sanskrit for "home of peace"), a healing center and educational retreat in Escondido, California, near San Diego [3, 4]. The center offered workshops on life, death, and transition, becoming a sanctuary for those grappling with terminal illness and for those learning to support them. In 1984, she relocated the Elisabeth Kübler-Ross Center to her own 200-acre farm in Head Waters, Virginia, which she renamed Healing Waters [1].

Dr. Kübler-Ross's personal life was not without its challenges. She and Emanuel Ross had two children together—a son, Kenneth, and a daughter, Barbara—born in the early 1960s [3]. The path to parenthood had been difficult, marked by multiple miscarriages that tested her faith and resilience [13]. Her marriage, additionally strained by her demanding schedule and relentless focus on her work, ended in divorce [3, 13].

In October 1994, tragedy struck when a fire destroyed her Virginia home [13]. The blaze consumed decades of her papers, diaries, case histories, patient records, her art collection, and most of her family's memorabilia [13]. Shortly after, she suffered a transient ischemic attack. She relocated to Scottsdale, Arizona, to be near her son, and the Elisabeth Kübler-Ross Center in Virginia ceased operations [3, 13].

In May 1995, she suffered a larger stroke that left her confined to a wheelchair [3]. For someone who had spent her life in constant motion—traveling, teaching, caring for others—this physical limitation was profoundly difficult. She found herself experiencing the very thing she had spent her career studying: facing her own mortality. In a 1997 interview with Oprah Winfrey, who flew to Arizona to meet with her, Kübler-Ross discussed whether she herself was going through the five stages of grief as she processed her physical decline [3, 13].

The irony was not lost on her, and she approached it with characteristic honesty and a dark sense of humor. In a 2002 interview with The Arizona Republic, she stated bluntly that she was ready for death and even welcomed it, calling God "a damned procrastinator [1]." Despite her spiritual beliefs about the continuity of consciousness beyond physical death, or perhaps because of them, she wished to have some control over when she would make that transition.

In July 2001, she traveled to Switzerland one last time to celebrate her 75th birthday with her triplet sisters, returning to the land of her birth and reconnecting with the women with whom she had shared that precarious entry into the world [1]. It was a journey full of memories—the mountain hikes, the flat rock, the war years, the long path that had led from that Swiss hospital where three tiny babies fought for life to international recognition as one of the most important thinkers of the twentieth century.

In her final years, working with author David Kessler, she completed one last book: "On Grief and Grieving," published in 2005, shortly after her death [3, 14]. With her two children at her side in Scottsdale, Elisabeth Kübler-Ross died of natural causes on August 24, 2004. She was 78 years old [1, 3, 4].

In 1999, 5 years before her death, Time magazine honored Elisabeth Kübler-Ross as one of the "100 Most Important Thinkers" of the twentieth century [3]. That same year, the New York Public Library named "On Death and Dying" one of its "Books of the Century [3, 4]." These recognitions acknowledged not just her contributions to medicine but her impact on how an entire culture thought about and dealt with mortality.

In 2007, 3 years after her death, she was inducted into the National Women's Hall of Fame, taking her place among the most influential women in American history [2, 3]. Throughout her career, she received over 100 awards, including 20 honorary degrees from universities around the world [3, 4]. In 2005, the American College of Physicians posthumously awarded her the William C. Menninger Award, and in 2006, the Hospice and Palliative Nurses Association awarded her their Medal of Honor [1].

Her archives found a permanent home at Stanford University's Green Library in 2019, donated by her family to ensure that her legacy and contributions to end-of-life care would be preserved and accessible for future generations of researchers, clinicians, and students [15]. The Elisabeth Kübler-Ross Foundation, established by her son Ken Ross, continues her mission, supporting end-of-life care initiatives and grief counseling programs in more than a dozen countries [1].

But perhaps the most remarkable testament to her influence is how thoroughly her ideas have permeated popular culture. The five stages of grief have been referenced in countless television shows, films, books, and songs. Shows like "Six Feet Under," "Bates Motel," and "The Good Doctor" explored themes of death and dying with a frankness that would have been unthinkable before Dr. Kübler-Ross opened the conversation [1]. Her model has been parodied and referenced in comedies like "Curb Your Enthusiasm" and "The Simpsons," proof that it has become part of our common cultural vocabulary [1].

In the business world, the Kübler-Ross Change Curve—an adaptation of her grief model applied to organizational change management—has become a foundational tool used by hundreds of the world's largest corporations. The framework helps employees navigate transitions, losses, and changes in the workplace, demonstrating how her insights into processing loss extend far beyond terminal illness [1].

In her 1997 autobiography, "The Wheel of Life: A Memoir of Living and Dying," Kübler-Ross summed up her improbable journey with characteristic wit: "I was supposed to have been a housewife. Instead, I ended up an opinionated psychiatrist who communicates with spirits from a world far more loving and glorious than our own [5]."

Returning to that question posed to my residency class, "What is the difference between a physician and a patient?" and the answer, "Time," I think about how Dr. Elisabeth Kübler-Ross understood this truth, and she used her time to transform how all of us—physicians and patients alike—understand our shared human destiny. For that gift, we remain forever in her debt.

References

1. EKR Foundation. Elisabeth Kübler-Ross biography. 2025, June 21. https://www.ekrfoundation.org/elisabeth-kubler-ross/biography/.
2. Women of the Hall. Kübler-Ross, Elisabeth. n.d. https://www.womenofthehall.org/inductee/elisabeth-kblerross/.
3. Bauer P. Elisabeth Kübler-Ross. In: Encyclopædia Britannica. 2022. https://www.britannica.com/biography/Elisabeth-Kubler-Ross.
4. EBSCO. Elisabeth Kübler-Ross | Research starters. n.d. https://www.ebsco.com/research-starters/biography/elisabeth-kubler-ross.
5. Kübler-Ross E. The wheel of life: a memoir of living and dying. New York: Scribner; 1997.
6. Wander Women Project. Elisabeth Kübler-Ross, 1926–2004. 2023, April 12. https://wanderwomenproject.com/women/elisabeth-kubler-ross/.
7. Newman L. Elisabeth Kübler-Ross. BMJ: Br Med J. 2004;329(7466):627.
8. National Library of Medicine. Changing the face of medicine. n.d. https://www.nlm.nih.gov/exhibition/changing-the-face-of-medicine/index.html.
9. The Independent. Elisabeth Kübler-Ross [Obituary]. 2004, August 27. https://www.independent.co.uk/news/obituaries/elisabeth-k-atilde-frac14-blerross-550364.html.
10. Blaylock BL. In memoriam: Elisabeth Kubler-Ross, 1926–2004. Fam Syst Health. 2005;23(1):108–9. https://doi.org/10.1037/1091-7527.23.1.108.
11. Kübler-Ross E. On death and dying. New York: Macmillan; 1969.
12. Paris JJ, Cummings BM. Elisabeth Kübler-Ross: a pioneer thinker, influential teacher and contributor to clinical ethics. Am J Bioeth. 2019;19(12):49–51. https://doi.org/10.1080/15265161.2019.1674549.
13. Bennetts L. Elisabeth Kübler-Ross's final passage. Vanity Fair. 1997, June. https://vanityfair.azurewebsites.net/article/1997/6/elisabeth-kubler-rosss-final-passage.
14. Kübler-Ross E, Kessler D. On grief and grieving: finding the meaning of grief through the five stages of loss. New York: Scribner; 2005.
15. Stanford Medicine. Stanford acquires archive of palliative care pioneer Elisabeth Kübler-Ross. 2019, March 26. https://med.stanford.edu/news/all-news/2019/03/stanford-acquires-archive-of-elisabeth-kubler-ross.html.

Chapter 2
Rita Charon, MD, PhD

I wrote my first short story when I was a little over 13 years old and have been jotting down my imaginary worlds ever since. Writing was as delightful as it was cathartic, and nothing could quite replicate the feeling of penning the perfect dialogue, the ultimate exit and the most arresting battle. Mystery, I could not quite enter, but Fantasy, Romance and Adventure were my playgrounds. Two Young Adult novels later, I received my acceptance into medical school. That long-awaited letter arrived in November of 2014, and I almost immediately plunged myself into any and all forms of media with a medical tint. From Grey's Anatomy ('e' not 'a') to essays written by current medical students on expeditions to international clinics. The latter I found on a website called "Aspiring Docs Diaries." At the end of the story depicting the life-altering interactions which a fourth-year medical student was privileged to have in Rwanda, there was the link asking for contributions. Aspiring Docs Diaries was run by the Association of American Medical Colleges (AAMC), and I was about to become their newest author.

At the time, I was a Research Study Assistant at Memorial Sloan Kettering Cancer Center and could shadow the oncology attendings on weekend rounds. I was a sponge as we traversed the halls of the inpatient unit; absorbing lingo I would not have the opportunity to use for years, and learning pathophysiology I quickly forgot, before I relearned it months later. And while I cannot confirm the academic value of trailing my mentors from room to room, there was much I could not fail to grasp about the human spirit in the face of illness. I witnessed my first code, my first discussion about code status, my first nighttime admission (yes, I even joined the nocturnalists overnight as any overzealous pre-med would) and my first sleep in a call room. I journaled every encounter and returned frequently to each essay to refine my descriptions of emotions—sometimes harrowing—which I had glimpsed. In a classic case of preparation meeting opportunity, I discovered the Aspiring Docs Diaries shortly after I began typing out my hospital encounters. My inquiry to them was met with warmth and, following some editorial work, my first essay was published. I was soon sending in an essay every month. As Fall approached and medical

O. M. Cox, *The Pen, The Stethoscope, and The Scalpel*,
https://doi.org/10.1007/978-3-032-19406-0_2

school drew closer, I was encouraged by my mentor, Michael Postow, MD, to prepare an essay for submission. Not to the AAMC, but to a journal, under the umbrella of what I would learn was Narrative Medicine. *On Rounds: The King* was born.

While I considered my writing for Aspiring Docs Diaries to be akin to blogging, submission to a journal represented joining the medical literature in a way that I had thought was reserved for only the most serious scientists. I, an almost-medical-student, could not possibly be a serious scientist. But when I investigated Narrative Medicine, I found Dr. Rita Charon and learned that the art of medicine was best shown in sharp relief by the written word.

Dr. Rita Charon was born in Providence, Rhode Island in 1949, in a world where medicine was not an abstract profession but an intimate, communal act [1, 2]. Her father was a general practitioner serving the French-Canadian population of the city, and from her earliest years, Rita was immersed in the rhythms and rituals of patient care [1, 3]. She would visit her father's office, often to sterilize equipment, and organize samples in the back room. The privacy of his consultation room was sacrosanct, but she could not help being aware of who walked through those doors; her religion teacher, the parents of the boy she had a crush on, the neighbors she saw at church. Medicine, she learned early, was deeply personal, profoundly human, and existed at the intersection of science and story [1].

Her father became her inspiration, though the path to following in his footsteps was neither straight nor immediate [1]. After graduating with a bachelor's degree in biology and child education from Fordham University's Experimental College in 1970, Rita did not rush into medical school [1, 4, 5]. Instead, she became a primary school teacher, drove a school bus, and threw herself into the peace movement of the late 1960s and early 1970s [1, 3]. It was 1968 when she started college, and there were, as she would later recall, "more important things to do than join one of the elite professions [3]." There was a war to be ended. The Vietnam War.

But eventually, medicine called to her, or perhaps she realized it had been calling all along. She saw becoming a doctor as an ideal way to teach, to learn, and to work toward peace and justice. It was also, she acknowledged, her way of paying tribute to her father [1]. In the mid-1970s, she enrolled at Harvard Medical School, graduating in 1978 [1, 6]. She chose to train at Montefiore Hospital's Residency Program in Social Medicine, which she considered the most progressive training available, and became a general internist dedicated to primary care [1, 3, 4].

In 1982, Dr. Rita Charon began teaching at Columbia University College of Physicians and Surgeons, initially as an instructor in clinical medicine [1, 4]. She also opened a practice in Columbia's medicine clinic, caring for patients in Washington Heights, a vibrant, multiethnic, predominantly Dominican neighborhood in upper Manhattan. For the next 35 years, she would maintain this dual identity: scholar and clinician [2, 7].

It was in her office, seeing patients every few months, that something began to gnaw at her. She found herself listening to her patients—really listening—and realizing that the stories they told about their illnesses, their lives, their fears and hopes, were not incidental to their medical care. They were central to it. But her training had not equipped her to fully receive these stories, to understand their structure and meaning, to recognize the narrative work happening in every clinical encounter [7].

When she mentioned to a mentor that she was thinking about taking a course in English, the mentor's response was immediate: "Rita, don't take a course, take a Masters [8]." It was the right advice. In 1990, while working full-time as a physician, Dr. Charon completed a master's degree in English at Columbia University [1, 3]. But one degree was not enough. She continued her studies, and in 1999, she earned her PhD in English, focusing her dissertation on the late works of Henry James and literary analyses of medical texts [3, 4, 9]. Her academic mentor was Steven Marcus, a renowned literary scholar who honed her writing skills [10]. Her healthcare mentor was Elliot Mishler, a sociologist and linguist whose studies of doctor-patient communication, helped underscore in her, that her passion and place in medicine was in its language [2].

The decision to pursue advanced degrees in English while practicing medicine full-time might have seemed eccentric to some of her colleagues. But to Dr. Charon, it made perfect sense. Every seminar she took—from contemporary poetry to Aristotle, from narrative theory to close reading—taught her something critical for the care of patients. She began to change how she practiced. She would put aside the chart, roll her seat away from the desk, put her hands in her lap, and say to each new patient: "I will be your doctor. Tell me what you think I should know about you [8]."

The results were revelatory. One woman replied, "You mean you want me to talk? [8]" The question spoke volumes about her prior experiences with physicians. Another patient shared, "Well, I didn't tell you about the fire in our house in Panama [5]," which turned out to be pivotal for understanding her condition. Others revealed, "I didn't tell you that my daughter is in prison [5]," or "I didn't tell you that I was in prison, but here, I brought you a book of poems that I wrote while I was in prison [5]."

Dr. Charon discovered that when she gave patients permission to tell their stories, they provided not just medical information but context, causality, and meaning. They revealed social problems that affected their health; the inability to afford medications, difficulty accessing care, and trauma that manifested as physical symptoms. They offered clues about their values, priorities, fears, and sources of resilience. And crucially, they felt seen and heard in a way that the traditional problem-oriented medical interview did not allow.

In 2000, Dr. Charon and some colleagues who were similarly interested in the connections between literature and medicine applied for and received funding from the National Endowment for the Humanities [3]. Other doctors and scholars nationally and internationally were exploring this terrain, but Dr. Charon and her team were the only ones who secured NEH funding to systematically study why teaching literary practices like close reading and narrative theory to medical students might be beneficial [9]. This grant would prove transformative [11].

With the funding, she assembled a remarkable interdisciplinary team at Columbia: professors of English, art, and cinema studies, along with pediatricians, psychoanalysts, and internists [3, 11]. Together, they developed a theoretical framework for what Dr. Charon would name "narrative medicine." The term appeared in her publication in 2000, formally coining a new field of study and practice [3, 10].

In 2006, Dr. Charon published her groundbreaking book, "Narrative Medicine: Honoring the Stories of Illness [3, 9, 10, 12]." The book was both a theoretical primer and a practical guide, weaving together insights from literary studies, philosophy, anthropology, psychotherapy, and clinical practice. It presented narrative medicine as "medicine practiced with the competence to recognize, absorb, interpret, and be moved by the stories of illness [3, 12]."

The book's central argument was both simple and radical: that by placing events in temporal order, establishing connections through metaphor and narrative structure, and truly listening to patients' stories, doctors could provide more humane, ethical, and effective healthcare. Dr. Charon described narrative medicine as emerging in response to a commodified healthcare system that had come to place corporate and bureaucratic concerns over the needs of patients. In an era of eight-minute appointments and checkbox medicine, she was calling for a return to presence, attention, and genuine human connection.

The response was overwhelming. "Narrative Medicine: Honoring the Stories of Illness" became essential reading not just for medical professionals but for anyone interested in healthcare, humanities, or the intersection of the two. It received praise from The Lancet, Perspectives, and numerous other journals. One reviewer called it "a compelling mix, backed by the unusual authority of a physician who is also a literary scholar [13]."

In 2016, Dr. Charon and a team of contributors published "The Principles and Practice of Narrative Medicine," which served as both textbook and field guide for the growing movement [14]. She also co-edited significant works including "Stories Matter: The Role of Narrative in Medical Ethics [15]" and "Psychoanalysis and Narrative Medicine [16]." Throughout her career, she has published extensively in prestigious journals including The New England Journal of Medicine, The Lancet, the Journal of the American Medical Association, Annals of Internal Medicine, and literary journals like Narrative and the Henry James Review. She formerly served as editor-in-chief of the journal *Literature and Medicine* [11].

One of Dr. Charon's most influential innovations was the "parallel chart," a teaching tool that has since been adopted by medical schools and training programs worldwide [1]. The concept is deceptively simple but profoundly effective.

Medical students and residents are already required to write daily notes in their patients' hospital charts, documenting vital signs, symptoms, treatment plans, and progress. The hospital chart is highly proscribed—there are specific things that must be recorded, in specific formats, using specific language. But as Dr. Charon explained to her students, there are things critical to patient care that don't belong in the hospital chart, yet they have to be written somewhere [1].

"If you're taking care of an elderly gentleman who has prostate cancer, and he reminds you of your grandfather who died of that disease, every time you go in his room, you weep," she would tell them [1]. That emotional response is important. It affects how you interact with the patient, what you notice, what you might miss. The parallel chart became the place where students could record their own reactions, their attempts to understand the patient's perspective, their emotional responses, their doubts and uncertainties.

Through the parallel chart, students learned to pay attention not just to pathology but to their own humanity and the humanity of their patients. They developed what Dr. Charon called "narrative competence [17]," the ability to acknowledge, absorb, interpret, and act on the stories of others. This competence, she argued, was as essential to good doctoring as anatomical knowledge or diagnostic skill.

The impact extended beyond individual practitioners. In focus groups and national surveys, patients consistently identified their top healthcare priorities as: the doctor-patient relationship, evidence-based medicine, and care coordination among specialists. Narrative medicine directly addressed the first of these, and indirectly strengthened the others by creating physicians who were better listeners, more empathetic, and more attuned to the full context of their patients' lives [1, 17].

In 2000, Dr. Charon founded the Program in Narrative Medicine at Columbia University [3, 4]. What began as a small group of interested faculty and students grew into something far larger and more influential than anyone might have predicted. By 2001, Dr. Charon had been appointed full professor [1, 4]. In 2009, Columbia launched the Master of Science in Narrative Medicine, the first graduate program of its kind in the world [18].

The MS program drew students from diverse backgrounds: physicians seeking to deepen their practice, writers interested in healthcare, social workers, nurses, chaplains, and activists working at the intersection of health and justice [18]. The curriculum included close reading of literature, narrative theory, creative writing, ethics, and practical applications in clinical settings. Students learned to lead narrative medicine workshops, to integrate narrative practices into healthcare institutions, and to conduct research on the outcomes of narrative interventions [1, 6, 11].

The program's success sparked a global movement. Narrative medicine is now taught throughout the United States and internationally. Universities in Europe, Asia, South America, and beyond have established their own programs, often in consultation with Dr. Charon and the Columbia team. The organization Narrative Medicine International brings together practitioners from around the globe, while the Narrative Medicine Alumni Exchange sponsors collaborative research and scholarship among graduates of the various training programs [6, 11].

Dr. Charon became a sought-after speaker, lecturing at conferences, universities, and medical centers worldwide. She delivered keynote addresses, led workshops, and consulted with institutions seeking to build narrative medicine education and practice. Her teaching extended beyond Columbia's medical students to include training for faculty, trainees, and students across 10 different health professions programs at Columbia through her role as founder and director of Columbia Commons IPE (Interprofessional Education) [6, 11].

The research backing narrative medicine also grew. Dr. Charon secured funding from the National Institutes of Health, the National Endowment for the Humanities, the Veterans Administration, the Josiah Macy Jr. Foundation, the Robert Wood Johnson Foundation, and other organizations. Her research projects investigated the consequences of narrative medicine practice, narrative's contributions to social justice and equity in healthcare, narrative medicine pedagogy, and creative and humanities interventions in clinical work [3, 4, 6].

The honors have accumulated over the decades. In 1987, Dr. Charon became the first physician to receive Columbia University's Virginia Kneeland Frantz Award for Outstanding Woman Doctor of the Year [1, 4]. She was named Outstanding Woman Physician of the Year in 1996 [1]. In 1997, she received the National Award for Innovation in Medical Education from the Society of General Internal Medicine [1, 4]. She was awarded a Kaiser Faculty Scholar Award, a Rockefeller Foundation Bellagio Residence, and a John Simon Guggenheim Fellowship, one of the most prestigious awards for scholars and artists in the United States [1, 3, 4, 6].

But perhaps the most significant recognition came in 2018, when the National Endowment for the Humanities selected Dr. Charon to deliver the Jefferson Lecture, the highest honor the federal government bestows for distinguished intellectual achievement in the humanities [3, 6, 9, 19]. Previous Jefferson Lecturers included luminaries like John Hope Franklin, Toni Morrison, and Ken Burns. Dr. Charon's selection represented not just personal achievement but institutional recognition of narrative medicine as a vital contribution to American intellectual and cultural life.

Her work has been recognized by the Association of American Medical Colleges, the American College of Physicians, the Society for Health and Human Values, the American Academy on Communication in Healthcare, and the Society of General Internal Medicine [3, 4]. She has held national leadership positions in many of these organizations, shaping medical education policy and practice at the highest levels [11].

The influence of narrative medicine extends far beyond awards and accolades. Medical schools across the country and around the world have integrated narrative medicine into their curricula. The Foundations of Clinical Medicine course at Columbia, which includes narrative medicine as an integral component, has become a model for other institutions. Students in these programs learn "everything except the biotech [11]," as Dr. Charon puts it: how to talk to patients, how to build therapeutic relationships, how to conduct physical exams with attention and respect, how to grapple with the ethical dimensions of medicine [11].

First-year medical students at Columbia now take courses like "Race Sounds: The Art of Listening in African American Literature," where they practice free-form choral readings of poetry and learn improvisational exercises in listening and responding [6]. As one medical student explained, "Narrative medicine reminds us that there is a story behind everything, and that what we see as doctors in a moment in time is a snapshot [7]." This awareness—that every patient encounter is a moment in an ongoing narrative—transforms how young physicians approach their work.

In 2018, Columbia University established the Department of Medical Humanities and Ethics, and Dr. Rita Charon became its founding chair [3, 6]. The department encompasses the Narrative Medicine program, an Ethics program, and one in Social Medicine, creating an institutional framework for the humanities to shape medical education and practice. To take on this leadership role, Charon made a difficult decision: after 35 years of seeing patients, she closed her clinical practice [2, 6].

The decision was bittersweet. For more than three decades, she had maintained her practice in Washington Heights, building relationships with patients over years and sometimes decades. She had witnessed their children grow, their health wax and wane, their lives unfold [2]. These encounters had not just informed her teaching and writing, they had been the heart of her work, the wellspring from which everything else flowed. But the demands of building and leading the department, along with extensive international travel for lectures and consultations, had made it increasingly difficult to provide the continuity of care her patients deserved.

Even without seeing patients, Dr. Charon remained deeply engaged with clinical work through her teaching and her students. As Professor of Medicine and founding chair of the Department of Medical Humanities and Ethics, as well as professor in the College of Physicians and Surgeons, she continued to shape how future generations of physicians would practice [3, 6]. She co-chaired the Division of Narrative Medicine with a circle of directors and associate directors, creating a collaborative leadership structure that reflected narrative medicine's values of shared authority and collective wisdom.

Her research focus evolved to examine the consequences of narrative medicine training, narrative's contributions to health care justice and equity, narrative medicine pedagogy, and the ways creative and humanities interventions could transform clinical work [6]. She spearheaded studies examining whether and how narrative training improved patient outcomes, enhanced clinician wellbeing and reduced burnout, and contributed to more equitable healthcare delivery.

When the COVID-19 pandemic struck in 2020, narrative medicine took on new urgency and new forms. Dr. Charon and her team quickly pivoted to offering online training sessions for healthcare workers who were facing unprecedented stress, trauma, and moral injury [5]. The creative writing workshops, close reading sessions, and reflective practices that had always been at the heart of narrative medicine became lifelines for clinicians.

"We've had a robust international response to these training sessions," Dr. Charon reported [5]. Healthcare workers from around the world joined online gatherings where they could step back from the relentless demands of the pandemic, write about their experiences, and share their work with others who understood. "The creative work they are able to do and the responses they receive from their writing is soul-building," Dr. Charon observed. An emergency department physician told her, "I was able to breathe for the first time all week at your session [5]."

The pandemic also highlighted many of the systemic problems narrative medicine seeks to address. As healthcare became increasingly corporatized and commodified, with electronic health records reducing patients to data points and productivity metrics pressuring physicians to see more patients in less time, the need for practices that preserve human connection became more acute. When skeptics told Dr. Charon, "Rita, but who has the time to do that?" in response to her call for longer, more attentive patient encounters, her response was unwavering: "Eight minutes per patient is not medical best practice. It is not. It is a combination of bureaucratization, corporatization, the neoliberal, revenue-first way of life [10]."

She argued that certain specialties, particularly palliative care, had successfully made the case to legislators and insurers that their work required more time, that the depth of engagement with patients at the end of life could not be rushed or commodified. If palliative care could secure that recognition, why not primary care? Why not all of medicine? [10, 12, 14].

Looking back over her career, Dr. Rita Charon has fundamentally transformed how medicine understands itself. Every clinical encounter is a narrative event. Patients come to doctors because something has changed in the story of their health; a new symptom, a troubling test result, a chronic condition that has worsened. They need help understanding what is happening to them, what it means, where the plot might be heading. Doctors, in turn, must be able to hear these stories, to recognize their patterns and themes, to understand not just the biological mechanisms but the human meanings of illness.

By placing events in temporal order, by recognizing beginnings, middles, and endings, by understanding metaphor and symbolism and the ways people make meaning through storytelling, physicians become better diagnosticians, better communicators, better healers. A patient who says, "I feel like I'm drowning," is not just describing dyspnea, she is offering a metaphor that might unlock understanding of her experience of congestive heart failure, her fear, her sense of loss of control. A physician trained in narrative competence will hear that metaphor and respond to it.

The parallel chart taught generations of medical students that their own emotional and narrative responses to patients are not unprofessional distractions but sources of insight. The elderly man with prostate cancer who reminds you of your grandfather is not reminding you randomly; there is something about him, his manner, his story, that has triggered that association. Paying attention to that response might help you understand what he needs, what he fears, how you can best help him.

Close reading—the careful, nuanced analysis of texts that is the bread and butter of literary study—translates directly to close listening and close observation in clinical encounters. When Dr. Charon brings a poem by Ross Gay or a passage from Toni Morrison's "Beloved" to a class of medical students, she is not trying to make them cultured. She is teaching them attention, teaching them to notice what is said and what is unsaid, teaching them to recognize patterns and themes, teaching them to sit with complexity and ambiguity.

The work has spawned a new generation of physician-writers, medical humanists, and narrative medicine practitioners who are transforming healthcare from within. They lead ethics committees, design curricula, conduct research, publish essays and books, and most importantly, sit with patients and really listen to their stories. They understand that in asking "What brings you here today?" they are not just eliciting a chief complaint but inviting a narrative act that can be diagnostic, therapeutic, and transformative.

Throughout her journey, Dr. Charon has remained remarkably open about her own struggles and doubts. She has written about the "relentless duty" of being a doctor, the way the responsibility never truly ends even when you are "off." The level of responsibility she feels, even in offering what might seem like trivial advice to a friend or family member, is steep. She does not romanticize medicine or pretend it is always fulfilling. But she also expresses a simple, profound hope: "I hope I can listen to my own patients in a way that helps them to feel confirmed and helps them get better [1]."

Dr. Charon has also been honest about the trade-offs involved in her dual identity as physician and scholar. When students write to her—two or three emails a week, she estimates, from complete strangers—saying "I can't decide between science and literature, I can't decide between medicine and a PhD in English," she understands their dilemma because she lived it. Her response is both personal and political: you don't have to choose [10]. Medicine needs people who can bridge these worlds. And the humanities need engagement with real-world problems and practices.

In returning to my own journey—from that 13-year-old writing her first short story, through my fantasy and romance novels, to my acceptance to medical school and my time at Memorial Sloan Kettering—I recognize the guidance of narrative medicine, which gave me permission to be both writer and would-be physician. Dr. Charon delineated the skills I had been developing through years of creative writing as not solely hobbies to be set aside when I put on my white coat, but as tools that would make me a better doctor.

When I submitted "On Rounds: The King" to a journal, I was terrified. I did not think I had the right to join the medical literature as a storyteller. But narrative medicine taught me that stories are not separate from science; they are how we make sense of science, how we translate data into understanding, how we help patients navigate the bewildering experience of illness.

Every time I wrote about what I had witnessed, I was engaging in the practice that Dr. Charon had systematized and theorized. I was creating my own parallel chart, recording not just what happened but what it meant to me, how it changed me, what questions it raised. I was learning, as Dr. Charon's students learned, that the act of writing about clinical experiences is not self-indulgent navel-gazing but essential reflective practice [20–22].

References

1. National Library of Medicine. Biography—Dr. Rita Charon. Changing the Face of Medicine. n.d. https://www.nlm.nih.gov/exhibition/changing-the-face-of-medicine/physicians/biography_rita_charon.html.
2. Duboff K. A champion of narrative medicine. Harv Med Mag. 2018, August 21. https://magazine.hms.harvard.edu/articles/champion-narrative-medicine.
3. Irvine C. Attending physician: Rita Charon. National Endowment for the Humanities. 2018. https://www.neh.gov/article/attending-physician-rita-charon.
4. Women in Medicine Legacy Foundation. Rita Charon, MD, PhD. 2011. https://www.wimlf.org/rita-charon-md-phd.
5. Quirk C. The healing, humanizing power of narrative medicine. Fordham Now. 2020, May 28. https://now.fordham.edu/fordham-magazine/magazine-profiles/the-healing-humanizing-power-of-narrative-medicine/.

6. Columbia University School of Professional Studies. Rita Charon, M.D., Ph.D. n.d. https://sps.columbia.edu/person/rita-charon-md-phd.
7. Glasberg E. Narrative medicine teaches doctors how to listen to patients' stories. Columbia News. 2023, June 5. https://news.columbia.edu/news/narrative-medicine-teaches-doctors-how-listen-patients-stories.
8. Boone A. At the crossroads of arts and medicine: a conversation with Dr. Rita Charon. National Endowment for the Arts. 2022, March 23. https://www.arts.gov/stories/blog/2022/crossroads-arts-and-medicine-conversation-dr-rita-charon.
9. Scanlan LW. Patient health through narrative medicine. National Endowment for the Humanities. n.d. https://www.neh.gov/project/patient-health-through-narrative-medicine.
10. Peede JP. Doctor of narrative medicine. National Endowment for the Humanities. 2018. https://www.neh.gov/article/doctor-narrative-medicine.
11. Columbia University Department of Medical Humanities and Ethics. Rita Charon, MD, PhD. 2020, January 27. https://www.mhe.cuimc.columbia.edu/narrative-medicine/bibliography/rita-charon-md-phd.
12. Charon R. Narrative medicine: honoring the stories of illness. Oxford: Oxford University Press; 2006.
13. Micco G. Listening to the story of medicine. Lancet. 2007;370(9594):1203–4. https://doi.org/10.1016/S0140-6736(07)61527-X.
14. Charon R, DasGupta S, Hermann N, Irvine CC, Marcus ER, Colón ER, Spencer D, Spiegel M. The principles and practice of narrative medicine. New York: Oxford University Press; 2017.
15. Charon R, Montello M, editors. Stories matter: the role of narrative in medical ethics. New York: Routledge; 2002.
16. Rudnytsky PL, Charon R, editors. Psychoanalysis and narrative medicine. Albany: State University of New York Press; 2008.
17. Charon R. Narrative medicine: a model for empathy, reflection, profession, and trust. JAMA. 2001;286(15):1897–902. https://doi.org/10.1001/jama.286.15.1897.
18. Harvard Countway Library Center. Rita Charon. Women in Medicine Legacy Foundation: Oral Histories. 2011. https://collections.countway.harvard.edu/onview/exhibits/show/fhwim-oral-histories/renaissance-women-in-medicine-/rita-charon.
19. Wasley P. Dr. Rita Charon named the 2018 Jefferson Lecturer in the Humanities. National Endowment for the Humanities. 2018. https://www.neh.gov/news/dr-rita-charon-named-2018-jefferson-lecturer-humanities.
20. Charon R. What to do with stories: the sciences of narrative medicine. Can Fam Physician. 2007;53(8):1265–7.
21. Charon R. Narrative and medicine. N Engl J Med. 2004;350(9):862–4. https://doi.org/10.1056/NEJMp038249.
22. Columbia University Department of Medical Humanities and Ethics. Our work at Columbia. 2020, January 29. https://www.mhe.cuimc.columbia.edu/narrative-medicine/our-work-columbia.

Chapter 3
Perri Klass, MD

Over the course of my training, I have had the opportunity to talk about my writing—why I write, what I write, when I might write next, and had I heard of Dr. Perri Klass. These questions usually came in the context of interviews, when parallels were drawn between me—aspiring pediatric resident—and Dr. Klass—renowned healer of children, Public Health Hero, and author. I *had* heard of Dr. Klass, through her work in Reach Out and Read, a non-profit organization which promotes reading aloud to children, starting at six-months of age. She was *my* hero, and it was an honor to even be thought of in the same sentence. Finding age-appropriate books for patients (and siblings) seemed a natural part of a clinic day in pediatrics; it is hard to imagine this was not always a universal practice. And the concept is the essence of pediatrics—a well-nourished mind, just as a nurtured idea, can grow to inspiring proportions. Dr. Perri Klass saw beyond the single seed of a reading encouragement program, to create a literacy movement which has granted over 20-million books to children.

Dr. Klass was born in Tunapuna, Trinidad, in 1958, far from the American medical centers where she would eventually practice and teach [1, 2]. Her father, Morton Klass, was an anthropology professor conducting fieldwork in the Caribbean, and her mother, Sheila Solomon Klass, was a novelist and English professor [1, 3]. The family would later return to the United States, settling in New York City and Leonia, New Jersey, where Perri grew up surrounded by books, ideas, and the expectation that writing was simply what people did [1, 3].

"I come from a family in which most people write, and publish (though no one makes a living at it)," Klass would later observe [3]. Her father went on to become an anthropology professor at Barnard College, bringing home stories of cultures and human behavior [3, 4]. Her mother taught English at the City University of New York and wrote novels, modeling the discipline and craft of storytelling [1, 4]. Her uncle was Philip Klass, who wrote science fiction under the pen name William Tenn [5]. Her siblings would also pursue creative paths; her brother David Klass became a

O. M. Cox, *The Pen, The Stethoscope, and The Scalpel*,
https://doi.org/10.1007/978-3-032-19406-0_3

screenwriter, and her sister Judy Klass a playwright, Truman Scholar, and Senior Lecturer of Jewish Studies and English at Vanderbilt University [6, 7].

In this household, where writing was as natural as breathing, young Perri learned to love both the written word and the act of observation. She wrote fiction in high school, college, and graduate school, developing an ear for dialogue and an eye for detail [3]. But she also inherited something else from her parents: a fascination with how people live, how they make meaning from their experiences, and how stories help us understand ourselves and others.

There was a moment in her childhood that would prove transformative, though she might not have recognized it at the time. In fourth grade, Perri had a teacher named Miriam Marecek who understood something fundamental about the power of reading. When Ms. Marecek wanted to share a story with her students, she would turn down the lights and light a reading candle [8]. In that candlelit classroom, magic happened. The ritual transformed reading from an assignment into an experience, from a task into a treasure. Decades later, as National Medical Director of Reach Out and Read, Dr. Klass would promote books and reading aloud to children starting at birth, carrying forward the enchantment Ms. Marecek had kindled in that fourth-grade classroom [8].

Dr. Klass graduated from Harvard University in 1979 with a degree in biology, but her path to medical school was not immediate or straightforward [2]. She spent time as a graduate student at the University of California, Berkeley, from 1979 to 1981, exploring her options [2, 3]. During 1981–1982, she worked as a researcher at the Institute of Parasitology in Rome—an experience that would later inform her decision to subspecialize in pediatric infectious diseases, allowing her to reconnect, as she put it, "in a certain sense" with parasites [2, 3].

But it was during these years between undergraduate and medical school that Klass began to crystallize what would become her dual calling. She worked as an instructor of expository writing at Harvard University from 1982 to 1983, teaching students how to construct arguments and tell stories [2, 4]. She continued writing fiction, publishing short stories that caught the attention of literary magazines. In fact, while still a student, her short stories won an O. Henry Award, one of the most prestigious honors in American short fiction [4, 9]. By the time she finished her career as a writer, she would win five O. Henry Awards, establishing her as a serious literary talent independent of her medical career [9].

In the early 1980s, Dr. Klass entered Harvard Medical School [1, 8]. She was in her mid-twenties, older than many of her classmates at the time, and she arrived with a writer's sensibility, a habit of observation, a compulsion to record, and a belief that stories mattered. What she did not know was that she was about to pioneer a new genre of medical writing that would influence generations of medical students.

In 1984, as a third-year medical student, Klass began writing a series of columns for The New York Times Magazine in their "Hers" column series [3]. These were not the sanitized, triumphalist accounts of medical training that had previously dominated the genre. Instead, Klass wrote with unembroidered honesty about the uncertainty of drawing blood for the very first time, the peculiar jargon of hospital culture, the emotional complexity of crying in the hospital, and the experience of being pregnant while in medical school [3, 9].

That last topic—having a baby while in medical school—became one of her most widely read pieces. At a time when women in medicine were still fighting for acceptance and respect, when the expectation was that serious physicians would delay or forgo family life, Klass wrote openly about navigating morning sickness between anatomy lectures, about finding childcare during clinical rotations, about the physical and emotional demands of gestating new life while learning to save lives [1].

Her columns resonated powerfully with readers, particularly with women in medicine who had felt alone in their struggles to balance professional ambitions with personal desires. But they also reached beyond the medical community to anyone who had ever wondered what really goes on behind the closed doors of teaching hospitals, what doctors-in-training actually think and feel, and whether the idealism that brings students to medicine survives the crucible of clinical education [10]. These columns and essays were collected in 1987 in Dr. Klass's first book, "A Not Entirely Benign Procedure: Four Years as a Medical Student." The title itself captured Dr. Klass's wry wit: honest, self-aware, and willing to acknowledge the pain and difficulty of medical training alongside its moments of transcendence [8, 9, 11].

The book became an instant classic. Medical students across the country recognized themselves in Klass's accounts of exhaustion, self-doubt, exhilaration, and occasional terror [9]. Here was someone willing to admit that she didn't always know what she was doing, that she sometimes made mistakes, that she cried in hospital stairwells, and that she questioned whether she belonged in medicine. And yet, she persisted, and in that persistence, she found meaning.

When Dr. Klass graduated from Harvard Medical School in 1986, she had already established herself as the voice of a generation of medical students [8, 9]. She completed her residency in pediatrics at Children's Hospital Boston from 1986 to 1989, then served as a staff pediatrician there from 1989 to 1990. She then completed a fellowship at Boston City Hospital in 1990, specializing in pediatric infectious diseases, a field that combined her early interest in parasitology with her commitment to caring for children [2].

During her residency, Dr. Klass continued to write, and in 1992, she published "Baby Doctor: A Pediatrician's Training," which chronicled her internship and residency years [8, 12]. If "A Not Entirely Benign Procedure" was about becoming a doctor, "Baby Doctor" was about becoming a pediatrician; learning to care for newborns, the chronically ill, and the mysteriously sick. It covered the acts of setting high standards for her own performance and for those who worked with her tiny charges, as well as navigating the particular emotional landscape of pediatrics, where every patient is someone's child and every outcome carries the weight of a future cut short or a life beginning [12].

Publishers Weekly called it "Riveting…An inspiring coming-of-age story and an inside look at medical education…A colorful, candid view of the exhausting, exhilarating and dehumanizing subculture of pediatric residency [8]." The book helped establish what has become a robust genre: the residency memoir. Today, countless physicians—including myself—have written about their training, but Dr. Klass was among the pioneers, showing that it was possible to write about medicine with both technical accuracy and literary grace.

The books were reissued in updated editions in 2010, introduced to a new generation of medical students. In the foreword to the new edition of "A Not Entirely Benign Procedure," Dr. Klass reflected on how medicine had changed in the intervening decades; duty hour restrictions, electronic health records, new technologies. She also chronicled how it had stayed the same; the fear, the learning curve, the profound privilege of caring for patients at their most vulnerable [8, 13].

But Dr. Klass was not content to write only about medicine. She had been writing fiction all her life, and she was not prepared to stop. Her first novel, "Recombinations," was published in 1985, while she was still in medical school [14]. It was followed by "Other Women's Children" in 1990, a novel about a woman who must balance her professional life as a pediatrician with her personal life as a wife and mother. The book, which drew on Dr. Klass's own experiences trying to "have it all," resonated so powerfully that it was adapted into a Lifetime TV movie [15].

In 2004, she published "The Mystery of Breathing," and in 2008, "The Mercy Rule," which The Boston Globe praised for its "breathtaking clarity and insight." In 2013, she collaborated with her screenwriter brother David Klass on a young adult novel called "Second Impact [14]."

She also published two collections of short stories: "I Am Having an Adventure" (1986) and "Love and Modern Medicine" (2001) [14]. Her short stories appeared in prestigious literary magazines and won five O. Henry Awards, a remarkable achievement for someone pursuing a full-time medical career [9]. The Washington Post noted, "As a doctor, Klass must know the body inside and out; these stories show that, as a writer, she knows the heart and soul just as well [8]."

Initially, Dr. Klass had thought she might keep her fiction separate from her medical life, that she would write about other subjects, other worlds. But over time, she found that her fiction became increasingly concerned with issues and stories that arose from medicine, from her pediatrician's perspective on the world. "Writers and doctors," she reflected, "have many overlapping traits; a fascination with the many stories out there in the world, an eagerness to probe for detail and complexity, a willingness to reformulate and retell. I suspect that by now my writing and doctoring 'selves' are profoundly intertwined, and certainly I hope to continue doing both jobs, with their particular challenges and satisfactions [9]."

Beyond novels and short stories, Dr. Klass's literary output included memoir, essays, and even writing about knitting. "Two Sweaters for My Father" (2004) collected her knitting essays, exploring the meditative, creative, and community-building aspects of the craft [14]. In 2006, she co-authored "Every Mother is a Daughter: the Neverending Quest for Success, Inner Peace, and a Really Clean Kitchen" with her mother, Sheila Solomon Klass [14, 16]. The book was a dual memoir, with mother and daughter alternating chapters, examining their decades of motherhood and daughterhood, the ways their lives had overlapped and diverged, their shared love of writing and travel.

Publishers Weekly called it "a treasure for any generation," and readers marveled at the intimacy and honesty with which the two women examined their relationship. Perri noted with amazement how closely her own life had mirrored her mother's: both had full-time careers (Dr. Klass as a pediatrician, Sheila as a college English professor), both had published books and stories, each had three children, both loved to read and travel. The act of writing the book together became another layer in their relationship, another way of understanding each other [8, 14].

In 2003, Dr. Klass co-authored "Quirky Kids: Understanding and Helping Your Child Who Doesn't Fit In" with fellow pediatrician Eileen Costello, MD [17]. The book, which addressed children with developmental differences ranging from Asperger's syndrome to sensory processing issues, became essential reading for families navigating the complex landscape of diagnoses, therapies, and educational interventions. A second edition was published by the American Academy of Pediatrics in February 2021, updated to reflect recent significant changes in recognition and care, with a stronger focus on self-care for parents and the pediatrician's role in supporting families through the diagnostic process [14, 17].

In 2007, Dr. Klass published "Treatment Kind and Fair: Letters to a Young Doctor," written in the form of letters to her older son as he considered entering medical school [14, 18]. The book addressed the fundamental questions facing any physician: expertise versus common sense practice, moral judgments on young patients or their parents, asking tough questions, death and physician-assisted suicide, the daily reality of a doctor's job, and what it means to be a doctor who is also a patient [18].

Although perhaps, Dr. Klass's most profound impact on medicine came not through her writing but through her work with Reach Out and Read. When she first became involved with the program, it was a single initiative in a single hospital. The concept was simple but revolutionary: at routine well-child visits, pediatricians would counsel parents about the importance of reading aloud to their children and would give the family a developmentally appropriate book to take home [19–21].

The idea addressed multiple problems at once. Many families, particularly low-income families, had few or no books at home. Parents often didn't realize how early they could and should start reading to their children, long before the child could understand the words, the act of reading together built language skills, strengthened bonds, and created positive associations with books. Pediatricians, for their part, needed concrete ways to support child development that went beyond treating illness [19, 21].

Through Dr. Klass's leadership as National Medical Director, Reach Out and Read grew into a national program operating in more than 4500 locations in all 50 states, distributing more than 6 million books every year to more than 3.8 million children. Dr. Klass trained doctors and nurses throughout the United States and internationally, including in Portugal and the Philippines, teaching them strategies to incorporate books and literacy guidance into pediatric primary care [19].

The impact was profound. In an essay about the program, Dr. Klass wrote: "When I think about children growing up in homes without books, I have the same visceral reaction as I have when I think of children in homes without milk or food or heat: It cannot be, it must not be. It stunts them and deprives them before they've had a fair chance [8]."

This passionate conviction drove her work. Under her leadership, Reach Out and Read became an evidence-based intervention with measurable impacts on language development, school readiness, and parent-child interaction. Research showed that children who participated in the program entered kindergarten with larger vocabularies and better pre-reading skills. Parents reported reading more frequently to their children and enjoying it more. The program became a model for how pediatric primary care could address social determinants of health and support child development in concrete, practical ways [19].

In 2024, Dr. Klass was lead author on a technical report published in the journal *Pediatrics*, the official journal of the American Academy of Pediatrics: "Literacy Promotion: An Essential Component of Primary Care Pediatric Practice." The report synthesized decades of research and clinical experience, making the case that early literacy promotion should be integrated into routine pediatric care, with counseling about interactive, developmentally appropriate reading strategies and provision of children's books at well-child visits [21].

Throughout her career, Dr. Klass has maintained her dual identity as physician and writer, each role enriching the other. As Professor of Journalism and Pediatrics at New York University, she directs the Medical Humanities minor, teaching students to bring together science and the humanities in ways that deepen both [10, 22]. She is also Co-Director of NYU Florence, the university's academic center in Italy, where she lives and teaches intermittently with her husband, history professor Larry Wolff [1, 13].

For years, she taught a course with her husband about children and childhood; he covering the history of childhood, she covering the biology and medicine. The place where their disciplines intersected was around questions of infant and child mortality and what it meant for society, family, and medical practice. This collaboration would eventually lead to Dr. Klass's 2020 book, "A Good Time to Be Born: How Science and Public Health Gave Children a Future" (originally published in hardcover as "The Best Medicine") [8, 14, 23].

The book told the story of how, over the course of about a century, infant and child mortality plummeted in the developed world, and increasingly in the developing world as well. Through most of human history, it was common for a third, a half, or even more of children to die before reaching adulthood. Parents lived with the constant expectation of loss. Culture was shaped by these deaths; diaries and letters recorded them; poets and writers lamented them. Even the wealthy and powerful lost children; presidents and titans of industry buried sons and daughters, though the poor and powerless lost theirs even more frequently [23].

But beginning in the late nineteenth and early twentieth centuries, everything changed. Germ theory led to better sanitation. Vaccines conquered smallpox, polio, measles, diphtheria. Antibiotics treated infections that had once been death sentences. Improved prenatal care, safer deliveries, better nutrition, and public health interventions all contributed. And for the first time in human memory, parents could reasonably expect their children to survive to adulthood. Early death became the exception rather than the rule [23].

This transformation, Dr. Klass argued, "is in no way a single project, but it can be seen as a unified human accomplishment, maybe even our greatest human accomplishment, at least for parents and pediatricians [24]." She wove together her own experiences as a medical student and doctor with the stories of pioneering women physicians like Dr. Rebecca Lee Crumpler, the first Black woman to earn a medical degree in the United States; Dr. Mary Putnam Jacobi, who fought for women's access to medical education; and Dr. Josephine Baker, who revolutionized public health approaches to infant and child welfare [23, 24].

The book was favorably reviewed in The New York Times Book Review and Library Journal. It resonated powerfully during the COVID-19 pandemic, when the fragility of public health gains became starkly apparent. As Dr. Klass wrote, the pandemic "harshly reminded us all of the fear and uncertainty that a new and untreatable infectious threat can bring [24]." The book served as both a reminder of how far we've come and a warning about how much we stand to lose if we abandon the public health infrastructure and scientific approach that made those gains possible.

Dr. Klass has been a columnist and contributor to numerous prestigious publications. She writes a weekly column, "The Checkup," for The New York Times Science Section, bringing pediatric perspectives to current health issues and helping parents navigate the avalanche of information (and misinformation) about children's health. Her medical journalism has appeared in The New England Journal of Medicine, The Washington Post, The Wall Street Journal, The New Yorker, Vogue, Gourmet, Harvard Medicine, and many other magazines and newspapers [8, 13, 22].

Her writing has helped medical students feel less alone, helped parents understand their children's development and health, helped the general public appreciate the complexity and humanity of medical practice, and helped physicians remember why they entered medicine in the first place. She has shown that it is possible to be both a rigorous scientist and a literary artist, that caring for patients and crafting sentences require similar skills of attention and empathy, that medicine is enriched by the humanities and the humanities are enlivened by engagement with medicine.

Her honors have accumulated over the years; in 2006, she won the Women's National Book Association Award, while in 2007, she received the American Academy of Pediatrics Education Award, recognizing her educational contributions that have had a broad and positive impact on the health and well-being of children [8, 10]. In 2011, she received the Alvarez Award from the American Medical Writers Association [8].

In 2016, the American Academy of Pediatrics honored her with The Arnold P. Gold Foundation Humanism in Medicine Award, citing the impact she has made through her writing, service as an educator, and leadership in promoting early literacy through Reach Out and Read [8, 10, 19]. The award recognized what colleagues and readers had long known: that Dr. Klass embodied medicine practiced with both excellence and compassion, that she saw each child as a whole person with a story, and that she had dedicated her career to ensuring that all children had access to both healthcare and the tools they needed to thrive.

In April 2021, Dr. Perri Klass was elected to the American Academy of Arts and Sciences, one of the nation's most prestigious honorary societies. The Academy, founded in 1780, honors individuals who have made preeminent contributions to scholarship, culture, and public affairs. In describing Dr. Klass, the Academy noted that she is "the leading journalist writing as a woman in medicine for the last generation," and praised her ability to bring together science and the humanities "in a unique and exemplary way [8, 25]."

She serves on multiple national advisory boards and councils related to children's health, literacy, and medical education. She has been a member of the National Institute for Literacy Advisory Board and the National Advisory Council of the National Institute of Child Health and Human Development. Through these positions, she has influenced policy at the national level, helping to shape how the country thinks about children's literacy, development, and health [8].

Dr. Klass lives in New York City with her husband, Larry Wolff. They have three children of their own, a fact she has written about extensively, examining the ways that being both a doctor and a parent shapes each role. In her book "Taking Care of Your Own" (1992), she explored the relationships between medicine and parenthood, focusing on issues like how doctors care for their own sick children. She concluded: "You will be the parent you are in part because you are a doctor, and you will be the doctor you are in part because of your children. Your medical career will shape their childhood years, and they, in turn, will shape you as a physician [3]."

When asked about obstacles in her career, Dr. Klass has been characteristically honest: "In many ways, I think my path has been pretty smooth; I have had great support, even when I chose to make my life complicated. The scheduling and the timing has probably been the greatest obstacle, especially when my children were small and there were long days and nights away, and often the sense of never quite catching up [3]."

That sense of never quite catching up is familiar to anyone who has tried to balance demanding careers with family life, creative pursuits with professional obligations, the desire to make a difference in individual lives with the ambition to change systems and policies. Dr. Klass has managed this balancing act for decades, and in doing so, she has served as a role model not just for physician-writers but for anyone trying to live a multifaceted life without sacrificing any part of themselves.

When I think about Dr. Perri Klass, I think about permission. Permission to be more than one thing. Permission to write honestly about the difficulties of medical training without being seen as weak or unsuited for medicine. Permission to have a baby in medical school. Permission to cry in hospital stairwells and then return to the wards. Permission to be a serious writer and a serious physician. Permission to care deeply about seemingly small things—a book given to a child at a well visit, a candle lit before reading aloud—because those small things accumulate into changed lives. Dr. Klass showed that it was possible to chronicle medical training without sanitizing it, to write literary fiction while practicing medicine, to advocate for public health interventions, and to find meaning in the daily work of caring for children.

As I moved forward in my own journey—aspiring pediatric resident, writer, someone trying to balance multiple callings—I carry with me the lessons of Dr. Klass's example. That writing is not separate from doctoring but essential to it. That observation and empathy are tools as important as stethoscopes and reflex hammers. That honesty about struggles and uncertainties does not diminish professionalism but deepens it. That giving a child a book is as much a part of pediatrics as administering a vaccine.

That fourth-grade teacher who lit a reading candle could not have known that one of her students would grow up to become National Medical Director of a program that brings the magic of reading to millions of children. Ms. Marecek could not have predicted that the enchantment she created in that candlelit classroom would ripple outward through decades and across the country. But that is the nature of teaching, of doctoring, of writing, of any work done with care and love; we plant seeds whose full flowering we may never see.

References

1. Hadassah Magazine. Profile: Perri Klass. 2007, December 13. https://www.hadassahmagazine.org/2007/12/13/profile-perri-klass/.
2. Prabook. Perri Elizabeth Klass. World Biographical Encyclopedia. n.d. https://prabook.com/web/perri_elizabeth.klass/637094.
3. National Library of Medicine. Biography—Dr. Perri Klass. Changing the Face of Medicine. n.d. https://www.nlm.nih.gov/exhibition/changing-the-face-of-medicine/physicians/biography_perri_klass.html.
4. Chicago Tribune. Young 'Superwoman' breezes through her whirlwind life. 1985, March 26. https://www.chicagotribune.com/news/ct-xpm-1985-03-26-8501170072-story.html.
5. Jonas G. William Tenn, satirical science fiction author, dies at 89. The New York Times. 2010, February 14. https://www.nytimes.com/2010/02/14/books/14tenn.html.
6. Vanderbilt University. Biography: Judy Klass. 2024, May 16. https://as.vanderbilt.edu/jewish-studies/bio/judy-klass/.
7. Breen A. This is who we are: David Klass. Columbia University School of the Arts. 2021, February 4. https://arts.columbia.edu/news/who-we-are-david-klass.
8. Klass P. Bio. Perri Klass, MD. n.d. https://www.perriklass.com/bio.
9. American Medical Association Journal of Ethics. Perri Klass, MD. 2000, May. https://journalofethics.ama-assn.org/article/perri-klass-md/2000-05.
10. The Nocturnists. The 100-year turnaround in child survival with Perri Klass, MD. 2024. https://thenocturnists.org/podcast/the-100-year-turnaround-in-child-survival-with-perri-klass-md.
11. Klass P.A not entirely benign procedure: four years as a medical student. New York, NY: Putnam; 1987 (Reissued 2010 by Penguin Books).
12. Klass P. Baby doctor: a pediatrician's training. New York, NY: Random House; 1992 (Reissued 2010 by Penguin Books).
13. GBH. Perri Klass, MD. n.d. https://www.wgbh.org/people/perri-klass-md.
14. ThriftBooks. Perri Klass books | List of books by author Perri Klass. n.d. https://www.thriftbooks.com/a/perri-klass/282318/.

15. Griffin D. Other women's children [Review]. Variety. 1993, October 20. https://variety.com/1993/tv/reviews/other-women-s-children-1200433600/.
16. Klass P, Klass SS. Every mother is a daughter: the neverending quest for success, inner peace, and a really clean kitchen. Ashland: Ballantine Books; 2006.
17. Klass P, Costello E. Quirky kids: understanding and helping your child who doesn't fit in. 2nd ed. Itasca American Academy of Pediatrics; 2021.
18. Klass P. Treatment kind and fair: letters to a young doctor. New York: Basic Books; 2007.
19. Reach Out and Read. About us. 2022. https://reachoutandread.org/about/.
20. Klass P, Needlman R, Zuckerman B. Reach Out and Read: literacy promotion in pediatric primary care. Pediatrics. 2003;111(3):677–9.
21. Klass P, Dreyer BP, Mendelsohn AL. Literacy promotion: an essential component of primary care pediatric practice. Pediatrics. 2024;153(1):e2023063518.
22. American Academy of Arts and Sciences. Perri Klass. 2021. https://www.amacad.org/person/perri-klass.
23. Klass P. A good time to be born: how science and public health gave children a future. New York: W.W. Norton & Company; 2020.
24. Reynolds E. Why we expect our children to live. NYU News. 2021, April 22. https://www.nyu.edu/about/news-publications/news/2021/april/perri-klass-on%2D%2Da-good-time-to-be-born-.html.
25. NYU Journalism. Prof. Perri Klass has been elected to the American Academy of Arts and Sciences. 2021, April 29. https://journalism.nyu.edu/about-us/news-post/2021/04/29/prof-perri-klass-has-been-elected-to-the-american-academy-of-arts-and-sciences-aaas/.

Chapter 4
Suzanne Koven, MD

I read "Letter to a Young Female Physician" some months into residency as a quick acknowledgement of a senior resident's recommendation, without fully imbibing of the lessons Dr. Suzanne Koven sought to impart. We too wrote letters to ourselves for future discovery, as had the residents at the opening of her letter. Unfortunately, despite the forewarning, I was doomed to recreate her residency story, until I revisited the letter near the end of my fellowship. Perhaps it is because those habits which seemed simultaneously to be the result of a "type-A" personality—so prized in medicine—and to be the mechanisms of survival in the sometimes necessarily harsh environment of residency, did not immediately scream out "imposter syndrome." Placing the obscure pattern on rounds and adding references to an assessment and plan could not possibly represent some kind of pathology. Until I examined the impetus for those behaviors. The problem was not the action, but the gnawing anxiety behind them which was identical to what Dr. Koven warned against. I've always believed that there is power in a shared identity and taken solace in the idea that I was not the first to examine a problem or encounter an obstacle. And while she was not the first to describe the phenomenon of "imposter syndrome." she did name our universal experience, and document the symptoms of this syndrome.

Dr. Suzanne Koven was born and raised in New York City, in a world where medicine was a familiar presence but belonged exclusively to men [1, 2]. In her neighborhood, the patriarchs were physicians—her father and the neighbors' fathers—while the matriarchs were mothers who baked kugel and brisket and acquiesced to their husbands. Looking for a snack in these homes, young Suzanne would see vials of insulin and penicillin lined up next to the chocolate milk in the refrigerator. Medicine was domestic and intimate, yet also distant and masculine, something practiced by fathers who came home late and talked shop at dinner tables [3].

Her father was a physician, and she would grow up watching him navigate the demands of medical practice. But unlike her friend Dr. Perri Klass, whose father's consultation room sparked an early fascination with patient care, Koven absorbed a different lesson from her father's career. She saw not just the intellectual challenge

O. M. Cox, *The Pen, The Stethoscope, and The Scalpel*,
https://doi.org/10.1007/978-3-032-19406-0_4

and the service to others, but also the toll it took—the long hours, the weight of responsibility, the way professional identity could consume personal identity [3, 4].

The women in her world, including her own mother, occupied a different sphere. Koven's mother was brilliant, but she was a housewife. Only in her 40s, driven by boredom and untapped potential, did she go to law school and claim a professional identity of her own [3]. This delayed claiming of intellectual ambition, would resonate throughout Koven's own life as she grappled with permission; permission to pursue medicine, permission to pursue writing, and permission to be both at once [3, 4].

Dr. Koven attended Yale University, where she majored in English literature [1, 2]. The choice was significant. At a time when pre-medical students were expected to focus on the sciences, when the humanities were seen as diversions rather than foundations for medical practice, Koven immersed herself in literature, in close reading, in the art of interpreting and creating narratives. She graduated with her B.A., but the path to medical school was not yet clear in her mind [1].

When she *did* decide to pursue medicine, she aimed high. She was accepted to Johns Hopkins School of Medicine, one of the most prestigious medical schools in the country, steeped in the tradition of William Osler and the history of American medical education [1]. She arrived in Baltimore with her love of literature intact but largely compartmentalized. Medicine would be one thing, writing another. She did not yet appreciate how profoundly they would intersect [1, 3].

Dr. Koven also completed her residency and chief residency at Hopkins [2, 5]. Here, Dr. Koven encountered a culture of excellence that was also a culture of stoicism. The medical interns called themselves the "Osler Marines," a moniker that captured both the pride of belonging to a distinguished lineage and the military-style toughness expected of trainees [5]. On one hand, being part of this tradition instilled in Koven a deep sense of pride and belonging to a rich heritage. On the other hand, as she would later reflect, she didn't stop to consider that the heritage was almost entirely male [3].

The internal medicine residency at Johns Hopkins from 1986 to 1989 was grueling. Residents worked exhausting hours, faced life-and-death decisions with limited experience, and were expected to perform with minimal complaint. The culture prized toughness above all else [5]. To show weakness, to ask for accommodation, to admit to struggling, these were seen as failures of character rather than reasonable human responses to superhuman demands [3, 5].

It was during this residency that Dr. Koven became pregnant with her first child [6]. The pregnancy should have been a joyous event, but instead it became a test of her belonging, her toughness, her right to be there [3, 6]. She was so determined to prove herself, so desperate to just belong and get through it, that she declined to request any relief from the exhausting schedule. She worked the same long hours, stood on her feet for the same endless rounds, pushed her body past reasonable limits [1, 3].

The price was steep. Dr. Koven developed preeclampsia, a serious complication of pregnancy that can be life-threatening to both mother and child. She was forced onto bed rest for the final weeks of her pregnancy, her body's rebellion against demands she had been unwilling or unable to refuse [1, 3, 6]. Looking back decades later, she would ask herself: "Why, as a pregnant woman, was I standing on my feet for hours, a factor that led to my developing preeclampsia? [6]" The question was not rhetorical. It cut to the heart of what it meant to be a woman in medicine, to the impossible choices and the internalized expectations, to the ways the system's demands could override a person's basic care for themselves.

After completing her chief year at Johns Hopkins in 1990, Dr. Koven joined the faculty of Harvard Medical School and began practicing primary care internal medicine at Massachusetts General Hospital in Boston [2, 5]. She would remain there for over 30 years, building a practice, teaching medical students and residents, caring for patients through decades of their lives [2, 4]. She married Carlo Buonomo, a radiologist who had also trained at Johns Hopkins [5, 6]. They settled near Boston and had three children. She later became a grandmother [5].

From the outside, it looked like success, prestigious positions, a thriving practice, a family, respect from colleagues and patients. But internally, Koven was struggling with a secret that she kept for decades.

Throughout her career, from medical school through residency and into her decades of practice, Dr. Suzanne Koven was haunted by a persistent, corrosive belief: she was a fraud. Despite her admission to Yale, despite her acceptance at Johns Hopkins, despite her successful completion of one of the most demanding residencies in the country, despite decades of excellent patient care and teaching, she believed that she was not smart enough or good enough to be a "real" doctor [3, 7]. She lived in constant fear that someone would discover the truth about her inadequacy, that she would be exposed as an imposter who had somehow fooled everyone into thinking she belonged in medicine [3].

This feeling had a name, though Dr. Koven didn't learn it until much later: imposter syndrome. The term, coined by psychologists Pauline Rose Clance and Suzanne Imes in 1978, describes a psychological pattern in which people—often high-achieving women—doubt their accomplishments and have a persistent, internalized fear of being exposed as a fraud [8]. Despite external evidence of their competence, those experiencing imposter syndrome remain convinced that they do not deserve their success and have fooled everyone who thinks otherwise.

For Dr. Koven, this syndrome manifested in countless ways throughout her training and career. She would overcompensate, overprepare, second-guess every decision. The obscure pattern placed on rounds, the extra references added to an assessment and plan, the staying late to triple-check orders—these behaviors looked like dedication and thoroughness to others, but they were driven by anxiety, by the gnawing fear that she didn't know enough, wasn't good enough, would be found out [3].

The syndrome was particularly insidious because medicine itself cultivated these feelings. Medical training is designed around hierarchies where students and residents are constantly being evaluated, constantly being put on the spot, constantly made to feel that they don't know enough. The Socratic method of teaching—where attendings ask rapid-fire questions designed to expose gaps in knowledge—can be pedagogically valuable, but it can also reinforce the feeling that one will never know enough, will never be good enough.

For women in medicine, these dynamics were compounded by sexism, both overt and subtle. Dr. Koven and her female colleagues faced harassment from fellow students, condescension from male physicians, assumptions that they were nurses rather than doctors, and a culture that viewed their very presence as provisional [3, 7]. While Dr. Koven notes that nurses were, in fact, especially supportive of the new women MDs—debunking a common myth—the broader medical hierarchy was less welcoming [3].

And yet Dr. Koven kept these struggles largely secret. She performed competence, performed confidence, performed belonging. She did excellent work. She cared beautifully for her patients. She taught her students well. But internally, she remained convinced that she was fooling everyone, that her success was a mistake or a fluke, that eventually the truth would come out [3]. It wasn't until half a decade later, that Dr. Koven felt something began to shift. She realized how much she continued to love writing, and how much she missed the intellectual engagement with literature that had sustained her at Yale. She began taking adult education courses in English, writing for fun, allowing herself to return to that earlier passion [3, 4].

Then, in a move that surprised even herself, Dr. Koven applied to and was accepted by the Bennington Writing Seminars, where she pursued a Master of Fine Arts degree in nonfiction writing [1, 4]. The MFA program was intensive, requiring sustained creative work, workshops where her writing was critiqued, and the development of a craft she had largely set aside during her medical training [1].

The program was transformative in multiple ways. First, it gave Dr. Koven permission to claim the identity of writer as well as physician. For decades, she had seen these as separate, even conflicting identities. But through the MFA program, she began to see how they could inform and enrich each other. Second, the act of writing became a way of processing and understanding her own experiences. As she crafted essays about her medical career, her struggles, her patients, her life, she gained clarity and perspective that had eluded her when these experiences remained internal and unexamined.

Third, and perhaps most importantly, the MFA program connected her with other writers; people who valued narrative, who understood the power of story, who saw writing as essential rather than supplementary to a life. This community reminded her that her love of literature was not a distraction from medicine but a central part of who she was.

In her 50s, Dr. Koven became a newspaper columnist and essayist. Her monthly column "In Practice" began appearing in The Boston Globe, where she wrote about medical practice, patient care, the healthcare system, and her own experiences navigating medicine and life [2, 9]. Her writing was marked by honesty, warmth, wit, and a willingness to be vulnerable. She didn't present herself as an all-knowing authority but as a fellow traveler trying to make sense of the complexities of medicine and human experience.

In 2012, her column won the Will Solimene Award for Excellence in Medical Writing from the American Medical Writers Association, recognition that she was not just a physician who wrote on the side, but a serious and accomplished medical writer [2, 5, 9].

In May 2017, Dr. Suzanne Koven published an essay in The New England Journal of Medicine titled "Letter to a Young Female Physician." The essay was framed as a letter to her younger self, her younger self as an intern 30 years earlier [7]. She had two things she wanted to say to that young woman, which she didn't realize until later were actually quite related.

The first was that 30 years later, there would still be sexism, misogyny, and lack of gender equity in medicine to an appalling extent. Women physicians still earned lower salaries than their male counterparts, were less likely to be promoted, more likely to experience harassment, more likely to shoulder disproportionate childcare and domestic duties [3, 7]. The progress that many had hoped for and expected had been slower and more halting than anyone wanted to admit.

The second thing, perhaps more personal, was about imposter syndrome. Dr. Koven revealed that she had spent decades—starting in high school, accelerating in medical school and residency—thinking that she was a fraud, suffering from what had been called imposter syndrome, though she didn't know the term early on. She wrote with devastating honesty about being "haunted at every step of my career by the fear that I am a fraud [7]."

The essay went, as Dr. Koven would later describe it, "as viral as a narrative piece in a medical journal would." It was accessed by thousands of readers around the world [4, 10]. Women physicians read it and found recognition. Men read it too, and some admitted that they also struggled with these feelings, though perhaps differently or less intensely than their female colleagues [4, 5, 10].

The response revealed something profound: imposter syndrome was not an individual pathology but a widespread phenomenon, particularly among women in medicine. By naming it, by describing it, by admitting to it publicly despite her evident success, Dr. Koven gave others permission to acknowledge their own struggles. She showed that you could be accomplished and still doubt yourself, that you could be competent and still feel like a fraud, and that these feelings, while painful, did not reflect reality.

The essay also drew critical attention. Some readers, particularly women of color, pointed out that much of what was being called "imposter syndrome" could be better understood as institutionalized misogyny and racism. When the system actively cultivates doubt in certain groups, when it provides less support and more obstacles, when it devalues the contributions of women and people of color, calling the resulting feelings "imposter syndrome" risks blaming individuals for systemic problems. One feminist scholar questioned, "Imposter syndrome? I thought we were all over that decades ago! [3]".

These critiques were important and Dr. Koven herself acknowledged in her book that while imposter syndrome is well-described and many practitioners identify with it, "it should be acknowledged that the system actively cultivates these doubts [3]." The question of how much to attribute to individual psychology versus systemic oppression remains complex and contested.

But what was undeniable was the impact of the essay. It started conversations. It brought issues that had been "hidden in plain sight" into open discussion. It connected isolated individuals into a community of shared experience. And it caught the attention of Jill Bialosky, a vice president and executive editor at the prestigious publishing house W.W. Norton, who wanted to buy an essay collection from Dr. Koven [1, 3, 4].

When Norton approached Dr. Koven about expanding the essay into a book, she was at work on a different memoir, one about her mother, whose heart disease she and other physicians had initially failed to diagnose [1]. The failure haunted her. "How much more of an imposter could I be," she asked herself, "than to fail my own mother in that way? [1]" The question captured the essence of imposter syndrome: taking a complex clinical situation, a diagnostic challenge that any physician might face, and turning it into proof of personal inadequacy.

When that memoir didn't coalesce into a complete manuscript, Dr. Koven accepted Norton's offer and transformed her mother's story into the emotional core of a different book, the essay collection that would become "Letter to a Young Female Physician: Notes from a Medical Life [1]."

The book, published in May 2021, consists of 24 essays that trace the arc of Dr. Koven's life in medicine. The essays are roughly sequential, beginning with her entry into medical school and ending with an essay dated April 3, 2020, "They Call Us and We Go," which provides an early glimpse of the COVID-19 pandemic and Dr. Koven's decision to volunteer for a COVID clinic after initially deleting the email solicitation [6].

The essays address the major themes of her career and life: pregnancy during residency in the AIDS era, the illnesses of her child (her son's epilepsy) and aging parents, the sexism, pay inequity, and harassment that women in medicine encounter, the near-universal challenges of burnout, body image, and balancing work with marriage and parenthood, and the inspiration she found in literature [3, 10].

But the book is more than a chronicle of obstacles and challenges. It is also a meditation on what makes medicine meaningful, on the role of empathy and listening in patient care, on the importance of storytelling, and on the search for authentic identity in a profession that often demands conformity. As one reviewer noted, "Koven's book invites us into her life and we discover ourselves in the margins [11]."

The reviews were overwhelmingly positive. Dani Shapiro, author of "Inheritance," called it "so wise, beautifully written, tender, and full of heart that it should be required reading for every person, young, female, physician, or otherwise [4, 10]." Andrew Solomon, author of "The Noonday Demon," praised Dr. Koven's style, wit, and grace, but emphasized that "more significantly," she writes "with insight and compassion [4]." Meghan O'Rourke, author of "The Invisible Kingdom," called it "a remarkable memoir about her life as a doctor that is at once heartwarming, poignant, and breathtaking in its precision [4]."

The Wall Street Journal described it as "a warm and wry epistle, the endless and near-perfect email you wish your mother, your mentor and your therapist would sit down and type out together [10]." The Association of Women Surgeons noted that "although the memoir addresses female physicians, I would agree with the many positive reviews that Dr. Koven's work is a 'Do Not Miss' for all genders, specialties, and disciplines in the medical field [4]."

The book found its audience not just among physicians but among anyone grappling with self-doubt, anyone trying to forge an authentic identity in a demanding profession, anyone balancing multiple roles and identities. Medical students devoured it and saw their own struggles reflected. One resident wrote: "I imagine that this is a book I could return to at many points in my career, and it would reveal to me different truths. I am reminded of the power of narrative, which is like a buoy in the ocean of medical training, bringing me up to see the horizon [4, 12]."

The success of the essay and the book coincided with a significant shift in Dr. Koven's career. In 2019, Massachusetts General Hospital named her their inaugural Writer-in-Residence, a position that Koven herself had designed [1, 13]. "I always tell people it is the coolest gig on the planet," she says [1].

As Writer-in-Residence, Dr. Koven runs a monthly "Lit Med" program in which a cross-section of hospital employees—nurses, doctors, administrators, and other healthcare workers—discuss literature ranging from Shakespeare to the South African novelist J.M. Coetzee [1]. The sessions are not about reading medical literature or discussing clinical cases, but about engaging with great literature and exploring what it has to teach about human experience, empathy, interpretation, and meaning-making.

Dr. Koven also coaches healthcare workers interested in narrative writing, helping them craft their own stories and find their voices. She mounts literary events, moderates panel discussions, and speaks to diverse audiences about literature and medicine, narrative and storytelling in medicine, women's health, mental healthcare, and primary care [1, 4].

Her conviction, born from decades of practice and from her own journey as a writer, is that "by reading literature closely, you become better able to elicit and interpret and respond to patient stories, which are foundational to providing excellent clinical care [6]." Reading, she argues, is "empathy in practice," and this is not "some touchy-feely add-on but fundamental to being a good clinician [6]."

At Harvard Medical School, Dr. Koven co-created and co-directs the Media and Medicine certificate program. She also serves on the faculty of the Media, Medicine, and Health master's program [2, 4]. In these roles, she helps train the next generation of physicians to think critically about how medicine is represented and communicated, how narratives shape understanding, and how storytelling can be used ethically and effectively in healthcare.

In recent years, Dr. Koven has significantly curtailed her clinical practice, not out of burnout or disillusionment, but to make space for writing, teaching, and her work as Writer-in-Residence [1]. She remains at Massachusetts General Hospital, where she holds the Valerie Winchester Family Endowed Chair in Primary Care Medicine, and she continues as an associate professor of medicine at Harvard Medical School [2, 13].

This shift represents a kind of permission she has granted herself; permission to focus on the work that feels most meaningful and urgent at this stage of her life, permission to prioritize writing and teaching over clinical practice, permission to be a physician who spends more time with words than with patients without feeling that she has abandoned medicine.

Her essay collection has been widely taught in medical schools and residency programs. Many programs have adopted it for book clubs and discussion groups. When Dr. Koven tours to speak about the book, she expects that the stories about sexism, macho medical culture, and difficulties combining pregnancy with medical training will be of largely historical interest to younger audiences. Instead, at event after event, young female physicians tell her that these issues persist. They describe inadequate accommodations during pregnancy, childcare and housework unequally shared with male partners, harassment, pay inequity, and imposter syndrome—all exacerbated during the COVID-19 pandemic—and how these factors have contributed to burnout and caused many to leave or consider leaving clinical medicine years before they'd planned [1, 3, 4].

The persistence of these problems is both disheartening and galvanizing. It means Dr. Koven's work remains urgently relevant. It stresses that the conversations she started need to continue.

When I revisited "Letter to a Young Female Physician" near the end of my fellowship, I understood it differently from my initial read, just months into residency. The first time, I had read it as a historical document, as someone else's story that might bear some superficial resemblance to my own, but that didn't really apply to me. I was fine. I was managing. I was succeeding.

The second time, I read it as a mirror. I saw myself in Dr. Koven's descriptions of overcompensation, of the gnawing anxiety beneath outwardly successful performance, of the constant fear of being found out. I recognized the mechanisms I had developed to survive residency not as signs of dedication but as symptoms of imposter syndrome. The problem, as Dr. Koven had written and as I finally understood, was not the actions themselves. It was good to be thorough, to know obscure patterns, and to reference literature. The problem was the anxiety driving those behaviors, the belief that I needed to prove myself constantly, that any mistake would expose me as unworthy, that my successes were flukes and my failures were the truth about me.

Dr. Koven's gift was in naming this experience, in documenting its symptoms, in showing that it was not an individual pathology but a shared syndrome that affected many physicians, particularly women. By writing about her own struggles with such honesty and vulnerability, she created space for others to acknowledge their struggles without shame.

She also offered wisdom about how to navigate these challenges. She didn't promise that imposter syndrome would disappear with experience or success, her own story proved otherwise. But she modeled ways of living with it, ways of building a meaningful career and life despite it. She showed the importance of finding one's authentic self rather than trying to fit into someone else's definition of what a doctor should be. She demonstrated the value of working part-time when children are young, of setting boundaries, of pursuing interests outside medicine, of finding community and support.

Most importantly, she showed that the solution to imposter syndrome is not simply individual psychological work, though that can help. The solution also requires systemic change: better support for pregnant residents, equitable pay and promotion, accountability for harassment, cultural shifts that value diverse ways of being a physician.

Dr. Suzanne Koven's career represents a particular vision of what it means to be a physician-writer. Unlike some physician-writers who wrote in the margins of demanding clinical careers, treating writing as a hobby or side interest, Koven has increasingly centered writing and narrative work in her professional identity. The shift from full-time clinical practice to Writer-in-Residence represents not an abandonment of medicine but a different way of serving it, by helping others reflect on their practice, by creating space for the stories that need to be told, by insisting that the humanities are not supplementary but fundamental to excellent medical care.

Dr. Koven is currently working on her second book, "The Mirror Box," a memoir about being a doctor who became a patient. The book will explore what happens when the person who has spent decades caring for others finds themselves on the receiving end of that care, when the interpreter of symptoms becomes the one experiencing them, when the doctor faces their own mortality and vulnerability. It is scheduled for publication by W.W. Norton in 2026 [4].

References

1. Johns Hopkins Hub. Holding up a mirror to a life in medicine. 2021, May 20. https://hub.jhu.edu/2021/05/20/koven-letter-female-physician.
2. Harvard Medical School, Department of Global Health and Social Medicine. Suzanne Koven, MD, MFA. n.d. https://ghsm.hms.harvard.edu/faculty-staff/suzanne-koven.
3. Koven S. Letter to a young female physician: notes from a medical life. New York: W.W. Norton & Company; 2021.
4. Koven S. About. Suzanne Koven MD, MFA. n.d. https://suzannekoven.com/about/.
5. Johns Hopkins Medicine. Beyond the dome: Suzanne Koven. 2022, November 7. https://www.hopkinsmedicine.org/news/articles/2022/11/beyond-the-dome-suzanne-koven.
6. Johns Hopkins Medicine. Hidden no more. 2021, October 5. https://www.hopkinsmedicine.org/news/articles/2021/10/hidden-no-more.
7. Koven S. Letter to a young female physician. N Engl J Med. 2017;376(20):1907–9. https://doi.org/10.1056/NEJMp1702010.
8. Clance PR, Imes SA. The imposter phenomenon in high achieving women: dynamics and therapeutic intervention. Psychother Theory Res Pract. 1978;15(3):241–7.
9. JewishBoston. Dr. Suzanne Koven is MGH's inaugural writer-in-residence. 2019, August 5. https://www.jewishboston.com/read/dr-suzanne-koven-is-mghs-inaugural-writer-in-residence/.
10. Harvard Mahindra Humanities Center. Suzanne Koven, Letter to a young female physician. 2021. https://mahindrahumanities.harvard.edu/event/title-event-suzanne-koven-letter-young-female-p.

11. Stanley MPH. Letter to a Young Female Physician: notes from a medical life by Suzanne Koven [Book review]. Intima: A J Narrat Med. 2021, December 22. https://www.theintima.org/book-reviews-intima/letter-to-a-young-female-physician-notes-from-a-medical-life-by-suzanne-koven.
12. Doctors Who Create. Book review: Letter to a young female physician. 2021. https://www.doctorswhocreate.com/book-review-letter-to-a-young-female-physician/.
13. Massachusetts General Hospital Giving. The healing power of storytelling. 2022, September 9. https://giving.massgeneral.org/stories/the-healing-power-of-storytelling.

Chapter 5
Lucy Kalanithi, MD

A little over a decade ago, in those 8 months before medical school actually began, I re-joined the platform formerly known as Twitter. I had worked as a Dell Representative in college and held the title of Social Media Guru for 2 or 3 years, while primarily managing Twitter accounts for Dell in the Northeast. Three years later I created a new account, @OMETrainingMD, and started posting content about my research and pre-medical experiences. This was the early days of #MedTwitter and as I found my medical niche, I was followed for it, by such impressive names as @MSKCancerCenter and @theNCI. I confess, I gushed the most when Dr. Carol Brown, Gynecologic Surgeon at Sloan Kettering, followed me, after my time shadowing her. #MedTwitter felt very much like the welcoming arms of medicine, and was the grapevine through which I learned about When Breath Becomes Air. There was a universality on that little blue social media app, via which we all connected with the shared purpose of medicine, while engaging with a mixed audience. We shared our stories, from awkward hospital encounters to research breakthroughs, from near death brushes to the steps taken to that inevitable path. I learned about Dr. Paul Sudhir Arul Kalanithi and his journey through the progression of lung cancer [1]. And then I learned of Dr. Lucy Kalanithi, who completed his words and story of the physician, who can become the patient and may become the caregiver [2].

Dr. Lucy Kalanithi was born in Paris, France in 1979, along with her twin sister, Joanna Goddard [2, 3]. The Goddard sisters spent their childhood moving between France, England, and Michigan, absorbing the cultures and perspectives of multiple worlds before Joanna eventually graduated from the University of Michigan and founded her lifestyle blog, A Cup of Jo [3]. Lucy, however, set her sights on medicine. She completed her undergraduate education and then matriculated at the Yale School of Medicine, where she would meet the person who would irrevocably change the trajectory of her life, both as a physician and as a woman [2, 4].

It was at Yale that Dr. Lucy Goddard met Dr. Paul Kalanithi, a brilliant neurosurgery resident who was, in her words, "unbelievably smart" and possessed a humor

O. M. Cox, *The Pen, The Stethoscope, and The Scalpel*,
https://doi.org/10.1007/978-3-032-19406-0_5

that made him "the funniest person I've ever met, while at the same time, soft-spoken and subtle [1, 5]." They fell in love during their medical training, two physicians learning together what it meant to care for the dying while simultaneously discovering what it meant to truly live. They married, both dreaming of careers spent in service to patients, both imagining futures filled with decades of practice, of research, of teaching. They moved to Stanford, where Paul pursued his neurosurgery residency and Lucy completed her internal medicine residency at the University of California, San Francisco, before returning to Stanford for a postdoctoral fellowship in healthcare delivery innovation at the Clinical Excellence Research Center [2, 5].

The future they had constructed in their minds—one of long careers, of growing old together, of watching their eventual children grow—was built on the reasonable assumption that time was on their side. They were young, healthy physicians in their 30s. Time, as that one visiting professor once told my residency class, was the only difference between a physician and a patient. But sometimes time collapses in an instant, and the difference between physician and patient disappears like breath on a winter morning.

In May 2013, during the final year of his neurosurgery residency at Stanford, Dr. Paul Kalanithi began experiencing symptoms that couldn't be ignored. Weight loss. Severe back pain. Chest pain that wouldn't relent. As a physician, he suspected cancer [6]. As a man in his 30s, a nonsmoker at the peak of physical conditioning, he hoped he was wrong. When a routine chest X-ray came back normal, he and Lucy allowed themselves to believe it was overwork, the physical toll of residency, perhaps early aging. But hope, as we all learn eventually in medicine, is not a diagnostic tool [7, 8].

The diagnosis, when it came, was as devastating as it was definitive: stage IV non-small-cell EGFR-positive lung cancer [1, 9]. Paul was 36 years old. Lucy was 34. In an instant, they transformed from a young physician couple planning their future to a doctor-patient-caregiver triad navigating an uncertain present. The neurosurgeon who had spent years learning how to save lives now had to learn how to live with death as his constant companion. And Lucy, the internist trained to care for patients, now had to learn how to care for the person she loved most while watching him slip away [8].

What happened next would change both medicine and literature, though neither Paul nor Lucy could have known it at the time. As Paul underwent treatment—targeted therapy that would give him precious extra months—he began to write [1]. He had always wanted to be a writer, had studied English literature at Stanford alongside human biology, had earned a Master of Philosophy in the History and Philosophy of Science and Medicine at Cambridge [1]. But medicine had claimed him, as it claims so many of us who harbor secret dreams of other creative lives. Now, facing his own mortality, he returned to writing with an urgency born of limited time and unlimited questions.

Lucy became not just his caregiver but his literary partner [10]. They would sit or lie side by side, Lucy sometimes reading Paul's words as he wrote them, the manuscript becoming a natural conduit for communication about what was happening, about how Paul was feeling, about what it meant to be alive in the shadow of death. "It was exhausting," Lucy later recalled, "but we were having a really good time. It was very purposeful; we loved each other and we loved Cady. We knew that Paul's time was limited and we were in pain [10, 11]."

Cady. Their daughter, Elizabeth Acadia, nicknamed Cady, was born on July 4, 2014, just days after Paul was released from a prolonged hospitalization [1, 9, 11]. In an essay for Stanford Medicine titled "Before I Go," Paul wrote about the joy his infant daughter brought to his life, ending with a message to her: "When you come to one of the many moments in life when you must give an account of yourself, provide a ledger of what you have been, and done, and meant to the world, do not, I pray, discount that you filled a dying man's days with a sated joy, a joy unknown to me in all my prior years, a joy that does not hunger for more and more, but rests, satisfied. In this time, right now, that is an enormous thing [12]."

Paul wrote with the discipline of a surgeon and the soul of a poet. His essays appeared in The New York Times, The New Yorker, The Paris Review. His op-ed, "How Long Have I Got Left?" articulated the impossible calculus of living with a terminal diagnosis: "The path forward would seem obvious, if only I knew how many months or years I had left. Tell me 3 months, I'd just spend time with my family. Tell me 1 year, I'd have a plan (write that book). Give me 10 years, I'd get back to treating diseases [13]." The piece resonated with millions of readers who had never faced a terminal diagnosis but who recognized the universal truth in his words: we are all terminal, all living with uncertain time, all trying to decide how to spend our days [9, 11].

As Paul wrote, Lucy cared for him with the unique perspective of a physician who loved her patient [11]. She understood the medical terminology, the progression of disease, the limited options available. She could read his lab values and imaging reports with the clinical eye of an internist. But she also had to live with the emotional devastation of watching her husband, the father of her newborn daughter, deteriorate before her eyes. In later reflections, she would acknowledge this duality, noting that even with her medical training, even with the support of family and friends, "it still took everything I had [11]."

Dr. Paul Kalanithi died on March 9, 2015, at the age of 37. He left behind an unfinished manuscript, a widow, a daughter who had not formed memories of him, and a question for Lucy: would she complete his work? [1].

The answer was yes, though it required everything she had left to give. Lucy took Paul's manuscript and worked with his editor to prepare it for publication. She wrote an epilogue that stands as one of the most moving pieces of medical and personal writing in recent memory [2, 11]. In it, she describes what Paul taught her about love, about presence, about choosing to move toward life even in the face of death. She writes about their decision to have a child despite Paul's terminal diagnosis, about the ways his cancer diagnosis became "like a nutcracker, getting us back into the soft, nourishing meat of our marriage [2]." She writes about watching him die, about the moment when breath finally became air.

"When Breath Becomes Air" was published by Random House in January 2016, 10 months after Paul's death [7]. It included a foreword by Dr. Abraham Verghese and Dr. Lucy Kalanithi's epilogue [8]. What happened next was extraordinary, even by publishing standards. The memoir debuted at number one on The New York Times bestseller list. It stayed there for over 70 weeks. It became a Pulitzer Prize finalist. It was translated into more than 40 languages. It sold over two million copies. Critics compared it to Joan Didion's The Year of Magical Thinking and Oliver Sacks's work. Kirkus Reviews called it one of the best nonfiction books of the century. Oprah Daily named it one of the best nonfiction books of the past two decades [7, 8, 14].

The book resonated because Paul had written it with brutal honesty and lyrical grace, asking the questions we all grapple with: What makes life meaningful? How do we face death? What is the relationship between doctor and patient when they are the same person? But it also resonated because of Lucy's epilogue, which provided not just closure but a different kind of hope; not hope that death can be avoided, but hope that love endures even when the beloved is gone. As she would write in a New York Times essay published the same day as the book, "My Marriage Didn't End When I Became a Widow": "Bereavement is not the truncation of married love, but one of its regular phases… what we want is to live our marriage well and faithfully through that phase, too [7, 8, 15, 16]."

That essay, like the epilogue, revealed Dr. Kalanithi's voice as a writer in her own right [2, 15]. Her prose is clear, unsentimental, yet deeply moving. She writes with the precision of a clinician and the vulnerability of someone who has survived unthinkable loss. She does not shy away from the hard truths: grief is not linear, widowhood is isolating, moving forward feels like betrayal. But she also insists on a broader truth: that love does not end with death, that the people we lose remain part of who we are, that we can honor the dead while also choosing to live.

Dr. Lucy Kalanithi could have retreated after Paul's death, could have focused solely on raising their daughter and practicing medicine. Instead, she chose to step into the public eye, to become an advocate not just for her late husband's work but for broader changes in how we approach mortality, suffering, and end-of-life care [11]. She began speaking at conferences and universities, appearing on PBS NewsHour, NPR's Morning Edition, Yahoo News with Katie Couric. She was interviewed by The Washington Post, The Wall Street Journal, Elle, The New York Times. She joined leadership boards for TEDMED, the Coalition to Transform Advanced Care, and the American College of Physicians [14, 17].

In 2021, Lucy launched Gravity, an award-winning podcast produced by Wonder Media Network that explores narratives of suffering and what becomes possible when we look at hardships differently [18, 19]. The podcast features deep conversations with thought leaders, personal reflections, and poetry. Episodes tackle topics like loneliness (with U.S. Surgeon General Vivek Murthy), the myth of the nuclear family (with Andrew Solomon), cancer metaphors (with oncologist Shekinah Elmore), climate crisis (with Mary Annaïse Heglar), and restorative justice (with Marlee Liss). In one particularly moving episode, Lucy revisits audio recordings of Paul to explore mortality and meaning, creating a conversation across the boundary of death that demonstrates how voices can persist even when bodies cannot [19].

The podcast, like her epilogue and essays, reveals Dr. Kalanithi's particular gift: the ability to hold space for suffering without being consumed by it, to acknowledge darkness while also finding light, to be both clinically precise and emotionally present. She speaks with the authority of someone who has lived through what many fear most, and she uses that authority not to provide easy answers but to ask better questions. How do we create meaning in the face of meaninglessness? How do we love knowing we will lose? How do we care for the dying while still choosing to live?

These questions have particular urgency coming from Dr. Kalanithi because she asks them not as an academic exercise but as someone who has embodied every role in the medical drama: physician, patient's family member, caregiver, widow, single parent. She has stood on both sides of the white coat, both sides of the hospital bed. She knows what it feels like to be the doctor with all the knowledge and none of the power to change the outcome. She knows what it feels like to be the family member who must make impossible decisions. She knows what it feels like to love someone who is dying, and she knows what it feels like to continue living after they are gone.

Throughout all of this, Dr. Kalanithi has continued her work as a physician. She is currently a Clinical Associate Professor of Medicine at Stanford University School of Medicine, where she practices internal medicine and leads innovative efforts to improve healthcare value and delivery. Her academic work focuses on patient engagement, shared decision-making, cost-saving innovations in stroke care, and improving communication between hospital-based and outpatient physicians. She has implemented novel healthcare delivery models across primary care settings, hospitals, and health systems [4, 14, 17].

Dr. Kalanithi has been recognized for this work with numerous honors. She is a Fellow of the American College of Physicians and has received the Stanford Medical Staff Awards and distinction from the Mass General Cancer Center's "the one hundred," which honors individuals who have made significant contributions to cancer care and research. These accolades reflect not just her clinical skill but her broader impact on how we think about medicine, mortality, and meaning [4, 5, 14].

Since Paul's death, Dr. Kalanithi has also found love again, a fact she has spoken about openly, recognizing that moving forward does not mean leaving behind. She is in a relationship with North Carolina lawyer John Duberstein, whose wife, poet Nina Riggs, also died of cancer. Their connection formed through shared grief: Lucy had corresponded with Nina and even provided a blurb for Nina's memoir, The Bright Hour, about her experience with terminal breast cancer. After Nina's death, John reached out to Lucy for guidance on grieving, and their friendship eventually became something more. It is a relationship born from understanding what it means to love in the shadow of loss, to build something new without forgetting what came before [3].

Dr. Kalanithi lives in the San Francisco Bay Area with her daughter, who is now in fourth grade. She describes Cady as funny, smart, full of life; qualities that echo her father. Dr. Kalanithi has worked hard to keep Paul present in their daughter's life, sharing stories and memories, making sure that Cady knows who her father was and how much he loved her. At the same time, she has created a life that is her own, that honors the past while also embracing the present and future [3, 10, 20].

The impact of Lucy Kalanithi's work cannot be separated from the impact of When Breath Becomes Air, the book she helped bring into the world. That memoir has become a touchstone for millions of readers grappling with questions of mortality, meaning, and what constitutes a life well-lived. It is required reading in medical schools and writing programs. It is given as a gift to newly diagnosed cancer patients and their families. It sits on bedside tables and in waiting rooms. It has inspired countless people to think more deeply about their own lives, their own deaths, their own relationships with time.

In her TEDMED talk, "What Makes Life Worth Living in the Face of Death," Dr. Kalanithi explores how suffering can be our greatest opportunity to love and be loved [10]. It's a radical reframing, turning what we typically view as life's worst experiences into potential sites of profound connection and meaning. She doesn't sugarcoat the reality of suffering, she's too good a doctor and too experienced in grief for that. But she also refuses to let suffering have the final word. Instead, she insists that even in the darkest moments, even when all hope for cure is gone, there remains the possibility of presence, of love, of meaning.

Dr. Lucy Kalanithi has not written a solo book, not in the traditional sense. Her primary literary contribution remains the epilogue to When Breath Becomes Air, along with her essay "My Marriage Didn't End When I Became a Widow" and her work on the Gravity podcast. But her impact on literature and medicine is no less significant for that. Sometimes the most powerful writing comes not from volumes of text but from a few thousand perfectly chosen words that cut to the heart of human experience.

Her epilogue to Paul's memoir does what great writing must do: it tells a truth that we recognize even if we've never experienced it ourselves. It shows us that love does not end with death, that grief is not a problem to be solved but a testament to what we've lost, that meaning can be found even in the midst of unbearable pain. It demonstrates that the physician's pen can write not just prescriptions and progress notes but also profound meditations on what it means to be alive, to love, to lose, to go on.

As I think about Dr. Lucy Kalanithi's place in this collection of female physician-authors, I return to that question my residency professor posed: What is the difference between a physician and a patient? Time. But Lucy's story complicates that simple answer. Yes, time separated Dr. Paul the physician from Paul the patient, and time will eventually separate all of us from our own mortality. But Dr. Lucy Kalanithi's work shows us that time is not just a separator; it's also a gift, a resource, a choice about how we show up for each other in the time we have.

Dr. Lucy Kalanithi teaches us, through Paul's memoir and her epilogue to it, that being a physician means being willing to accompany our patients all the way to the end, even when we cannot offer cure. She shows us that the work of medicine is not just about diagnosis and treatment but about being present with suffering, about helping people find meaning even in circumstances that seem meaningless. She evinces the truth, that love persists beyond death, that grief is not something to be cured but something to be lived with, that it is possible to honor the past while also choosing to live fully in the present.

References

1. Stanford Daily. Stanford neurosurgeon and writer Paul Kalanithi dies at 37. 2015, March 21. https://stanforddaily.com/2015/03/21/stanford-neurosurgeon-and-writer-paul-kalanithi-dies-at-37/.
2. Elle. When breath becomes air—Lucy and Paul Kalanithi. 2016, January 7. https://www.elle.com/culture/books/a32705/when-breath-becomes-air/.
3. Cup of Jo. Visiting my twin sister in California. 2023, May 30. https://cupofjo.com/2023/05/30/visiting-my-twin-sister-in-california/.
4. Stanford Profiles. Lucy (Goddard) Kalanithi. n.d. https://profiles.stanford.edu/lucy-kalanithi.
5. AAE Speakers Bureau. Dr. Lucy Kalanithi. n.d. https://www.aaespeakers.com/keynote-speakers/dr-lucy-kalanithi.
6. ABC7 San Francisco. Stanford neurosurgeon Paul Kalanithi dies from lung cancer at 37. 2015, March 23. https://abc7news.com/neurosurgeon-paul-kalanithi-cancer-patient/557650/.
7. Kalanithi P. When breath becomes air. Random House; New York, NY. 2016.
8. Kalanithi L. Epilogue. In: Kalanithi IP, editor. When breath becomes air. Random House; New York, NY. 2016. p. 195–221.
9. The ASCO Post. Remembering neurosurgeon and writer Paul Kalanithi, MD. n.d. https://ascopost.com/issues/april-10-2015/remembering-neurosurgeon-and-writer-paul-kalanithi-md/.
10. TEDMED. Lucy Kalanithi: what makes life worth living in the face of death. n.d. https://www.tedmed.com/talk/what-makes-life-worth-living-in-the-face-of-death/.
11. Cancer Today. Honoring life in death. 2018, Summer. https://www.cancertodaymag.org/summer2018/honoring-life-in-death/.
12. Kalanithi P. Before I go. Stanford Medicine. 2015, Spring.
13. Kalanithi P. How long have I got left? The New York Times. 2014, January 24.
14. Kalanithi L. Dr. Lucy Kalanithi. Lucy Kalanithi MD. n.d. https://lucykalanithi.com/.
15. Kalanithi L. My marriage didn't end when I became a widow. The New York Times. 2016, January 19.
16. NBC Bay Area. Late Stanford neurosurgeon's book about life, death receives rave review in New York Times. 2016, January 6. https://www.nbcbayarea.com/news/local/paul-kalanithi-stanford-neurosurgeon-book-about-life-and-death-receives-rave-reviews/141731/.
17. Aspen Ideas. Lucy Kalanithi: Clinical Associate Professor of Medicine, Stanford University School of Medicine. n.d. https://www.aspenideas.org/speakers/lucy-kalanithi.
18. Wonder Media Network. Gravity. 2021. https://wondermedianetwork.com/work/gravity/.
19. Apple Podcasts. Gravity [Audio podcast]. 2021. https://podcasts.apple.com/us/podcast/gravity/id1567923973.
20. Inside Edition. Sister surprises her widowed twin with home makeover. 2016, March 28. https://www.insideedition.com/headlines/15509-sister-surprises-her-widowed-twin-with-home-makeover.

Chapter 6
Rana Awdish, MD

One of the unique benefits of #MedTwitter, was the discovery that amongst those enduring the same vicissitudes in medicine, and celebrating the same victories over pathology, more than a few have straddled the fine line between patient and physician practitioner. We have winced at the undrawn curtains that turned our ICU room into a fishbowl, have groaned at the midnight awakening for vital signs whose meaning we tried not to interpret, or have witnessed rounds from the bed while *our* loved ones tried to follow along. I found Dr. Awdish's book, "In Shock: My Journey from Death to Recovery and the Redemptive Power of Hope," very shortly after I was discharged from the hospital, and coincidentally after I resumed my rotation in the PICU. I had been admitted for angioedema, with airway swelling requiring monitoring, but had been spared a prolonged hospitalization after a course of steroids. Our fellow at the time recounted her stint in the adult ICU following a challenging birthing experience, and our attending offered his tale admission for respiratory compromise. They both, then, recommended Dr. Rana Awdish's work, as a poignant reflection of our shared experience as physicians who had been struck with pathology. As was my wont, I found her on Twitter and immediately followed, to discover her love of her children's art, her penchant for painting and her talent for storytelling.

Dr. Rana Awdish was born in Michigan, a place that would become both the setting of her medical training and the site of her near-death [1]. She completed her undergraduate degree at the University of Michigan in Ann Arbor, studying biology [1, 2]. Like so many of us who eventually find our way to medicine, she was drawn by a desire to understand the intricate workings of the human body, to master the science of healing, to become the kind of physician who could save lives. She pursued a Master's degree in Basic Medical Sciences at Wayne State University before matriculating at Wayne State University School of Medicine, where she earned her Doctor of Medicine degree in 2002 [3]. At Wayne State, she was inducted into the Alpha Omega Alpha national medical honor society, a recognition that marked her as one of the brightest among her peers [1, 3, 4].

O. M. Cox, *The Pen, The Stethoscope, and The Scalpel*, https://doi.org/10.1007/978-3-032-19406-0_6

After medical school, Dr. Awdish moved to New York to complete her internal medicine residency at Mount Sinai Beth Israel in Manhattan from 2002 to 2005 [1]. The city, with its endless stream of patients and pathology, provided the kind of intensive training that shapes physicians into confident clinicians. She learned to think on her feet, to triage efficiently, to make decisions under pressure. She learned, as we all do during residency, to compartmentalize; to see the patient in the bed but also the disease on the chart, to feel compassion but also maintain the emotional distance necessary to function in the face of constant suffering and death.

Following her residency, Dr. Awdish returned to Michigan to complete her fellowship in Pulmonary Disease and Critical Care Medicine at Henry Ford Hospital from 2005 to 2008 [2]. She chose pulmonary and critical care because, as she would later explain, "it felt like the most concentrated form of internal medicine, where all the organs were accounted for and I could be present for the most critical moments in someone's life [5]." It was the medicine of extremes, where the interventions were dramatic and the stakes were life and death. In the ICU, every decision mattered. Every medication, every setting on the ventilator, every fluid bolus could mean the difference between survival and death.

She was good at it. More than good, she was excellent. Her training prepared her to manage the sickest of the sick, to remain calm in crisis, to execute the protocols that would save lives. She joined the faculty at Henry Ford Hospital and quickly established herself as a skilled intensivist and pulmonologist. She was on the path to becoming exactly the kind of physician she had always wanted to be: competent, confident, capable of extraordinary clinical feats.

And then, on the last day of her fellowship in 2008, everything changed.

Dr. Awdish was 7 months pregnant with her first child. She and her husband Randy had gone out for a celebratory dinner with friends to mark the end of her fellowship training [6]. They were celebrating not just the completion of years of arduous medical education but also the beginning of their family. The future seemed to stretch out before them, full of promise and possibility. And then, at the restaurant, Dr. Awdish experienced excruciating abdominal pain in her right upper quadrant. It came on suddenly, violently, with an intensity that told her immediately something was catastrophically wrong [6].

As a physician, she knew. The location of the pain, the severity, the sudden onset; these were not good signs. Her medical training kicked in even as her body went into crisis. She knew she needed a trauma center. She knew she needed it now. Her husband rushed her to Henry Ford Hospital, the very place where she worked, where she knew the hallways and the protocols, where she should have felt safe [6].

But being a patient, she would discover, was nothing like being a physician. At the emergency room entrance, a security guard triaged her. Not to the Level I trauma center she knew she needed, but to labor and delivery, because she was pregnant. Even though she was a physician at that hospital, even though she knew the triage was wrong, she didn't advocate for herself. She had already begun to learn what she would spend the next months discovering in increasingly painful ways: that as a patient, you lose agency with astonishing speed. When you're in crisis, when you're afraid, when you're in pain, you simply obey what the authority figures tell you, even when you know better [6].

In labor and delivery, a resident arrived who seemed uncertain, who fumbled with the ultrasound trying to locate the baby. Dr. Awdish watched from the other side—no longer the confident physician but the vulnerable patient—and saw what it looked like to be so unsure of your place in medicine. She was hemorrhaging internally, her hemoglobin dropping precipitously, but the focus remained on the pregnancy, on finding the fetal heartbeat, on determining the baby's status.

What Dr. Awdish didn't know yet was that she had a hepatic adenoma—a benign tumor in her liver—that had ruptured. She was bleeding into her abdomen, losing her entire blood volume into the space where it could do nothing but kill her. By the time she was rushed into surgery, her hemoglobin was three. Her platelets were 15. Her liver enzymes were in the tens of thousands. She was in refractory hemorrhagic shock with multi-system organ failure [6].

The baby didn't survive. Dr. Awdish nearly didn't either [6].

That first surgery was not the end but the beginning of a months-long ordeal. There would be multiple surgeries, multiple ICU stays, multiple near-death experiences. She would spend weeks on a ventilator, would suffer a stroke, would endure organ failure after organ failure. She would lie in a hospital bed in her own institution and overhear a resident say during rounds, "She's been trying to die on us [6]," as if her struggle to survive was somehow an inconvenience, a failure of will rather than a testament to her fight for life [1, 7].

The words struck her with particular force because she recognized them. She had used that exact phrase herself to describe her own patients in the past. "She's trying to die on us." As if dying were something patients did to physicians rather than something that happened to human beings. As if death were a choice, a giving up, rather than sometimes the inevitable end of a disease process despite everyone's best efforts.

Dr. Awdish lay in that bed, fighting for every breath, enduring unimaginable pain and loss, and she began to see medicine from an entirely different perspective. She saw what she had been doing, what all physicians are trained to do: to focus on the disease rather than the person, to prioritize the data in the computer over the human suffering in the bed, to maintain an emotional distance that feels like professionalism but can manifest as cruelty [6].

She experienced, firsthand, the casual disregard, not because her physicians were bad people, but because they were well-trained physicians doing exactly what they had been taught to do. They were competent, skilled, capable of extraordinary interventions. They saved her life, multiple times. And yet, alongside that technical excellence, there was an absence of something essential. A failure to see her as a whole person. A reluctance to acknowledge suffering. An emotional distance that, from the patient side, felt like abandonment [6, 8].

In the operating room, she was conscious enough to hear the surgeons talking about her as if she weren't there, as if the body on the table were just a body and not a person who could hear and understand and feel the weight of their words. They spoke in clinical terms about her deteriorating condition, about the challenges of the surgery, about whether she would survive. She heard someone say she was "circling the drain," another phrase she had used herself, another bit of dark humor that physicians use to cope with the emotional toll of caring for the dying, but which sounds very different when you are the one supposedly circling [6].

Through the weeks and months of her recovery, Dr. Awdish underwent a profound transformation. The physical healing was arduous; the multiple surgeries, the physical therapy to regain the ability to walk, the slow rebuilding of organ function. But the psychological and spiritual transformation was even more profound. She came to understand what she had been missing in her practice of medicine, what she hadn't been taught in medical school or residency or fellowship [6, 8].

"Despite completing my training," she would later write, "despite being surrounded by every form and severity of disease, I had yet to learn what it meant to be sick [6]."

She discovered that suffering is not just a symptom to be managed or a problem to be solved. Suffering is a profoundly human experience that requires acknowledgment, presence, and witness. Patients don't just need correct diagnoses and appropriate treatments, though they certainly need those. They also need to be seen as whole people, to have their suffering acknowledged, to feel that their physicians are present with them in their fear and pain and uncertainty [5, 6].

She learned that the emotional distance physicians maintain—the protective barrier we construct between ourselves and our patients' suffering—doesn't actually protect us from burnout or moral distress. Instead, it contributes to it. When we disconnect from our patients' humanity, we also disconnect from our own. We become, in Dr. Awdish's words, "ill-equipped to deal with suffering when it was in front of us," finding it "much easier to tend to the version of the patient who lived in the computer and not in the bed. The computer is neat and organized and has data. The person in the bed is messy [6]."

In 2012, 4 years after her near-death experience, Dr. Awdish started a communication program at Henry Ford Hospital called CLEAR (Connect, Listen, Empathize, Align, Respect) [2, 7]. The program trains medical residents, fellows, and faculty in relationship-based compassionate communication skills, using improvisational actors to help physicians practice difficult conversations and learn how to be present with suffering [6, 7]. It started as a one-department initiative and has grown into a system-wide program that has transformed the culture of care at Henry Ford Health System [2, 7].

The program addresses a fundamental flaw in medical education: we teach physicians the science of medicine but not the art of being present with another human being's suffering. We teach diagnosis and treatment protocols but not how to have honest conversations about prognosis and limitations. We teach emotional distance as a professional virtue without recognizing that connection—genuine human connection—is actually what allows both patients and physicians to survive the hardest parts of medicine.

Dr. Awdish became the Medical Director of Care Experience for Henry Ford Health System, a role that allows her to integrate compassionate communication strategies and narrative medicine practices into the curriculum across the entire system [1, 2]. She lectures to physicians, hospital leadership, and medical schools around the country, sharing her story and advocating for a fundamental shift in how we practice medicine.

And then she wrote the book.

"In Shock: My Journey from Death to Recovery and the Redemptive Power of Hope" was published in 2018 by Penguin Random House [1, 6]. The memoir is a hauntingly personal account of Dr. Awdish's catastrophic illness and her subsequent transformation. The book is unvarnished in its portrayal of both the medical system's failures and Dr. Awdish's own complicity in those failures. She doesn't present herself as a victim or a hero but as a flawed human being who, through suffering, came to understand fundamental truths about healing and connection.

The book is beautifully written, with prose that manages to be both clinically precise and deeply resonant. Dr. Awdish has a gift for metaphor, for capturing abstract feelings in concrete language. She writes about her experience of hemorrhagic shock, of organ failure, of near-death, with the kind of intricate detail that makes readers feel they are there with her in that hospital bed. But she also writes about the more subtle experiences: the loss of agency, the fear of being unseen, the existential terror of realizing that your body can betray you without warning, that all the certainties you built your life upon were illusions.

The book's timeline is intentionally disorienting, jumping back and forth in ways that mirror Dr. Awdish's experience of being heavily sedated, of losing chunks of time, of not knowing how long she'd been unconscious or what had happened while she was gone. Some reviewers criticized this aspect of the book, but Dr. Awdish was deliberate in her choice. "That was very intentional," she explained in interviews, "because I wasn't clear how much time I was missing. I wasn't clear when I would leave and come back what had happened, it was a very real uncertainty for me, and I didn't feel like it would be true to portray it as if it were just this linear timeline that made sense [9]."

The book became a Los Angeles Times bestseller and received widespread critical acclaim [6]. The New York Times Book Review wrote: "Awdish's book is the one I wished we were given as assigned reading our first year of medical school, alongside our white coats and stethoscopes…dramatic, engaging and instructive [1, 6]." Publishers Weekly called it "a compassionate and critical look at medicine and illness from both a doctor's and a patient's perspective [1]." Kirkus Reviews described it as "a sobering, well-rendered reality check on the desperate need for advanced training on compassion-centric modes of patient care [1, 6]."

Most significantly, the book has been adopted into medical school curricula across the United States and the United Kingdom. Wayne State University School of Medicine, where Dr. Awdish trained, is among the many institutions that now require students to read "In Shock." The book has become essential reading for anyone entering medicine, a powerful counterweight to the traditional medical education that prioritizes technical skill over human connection [3].

Dr. Awdish's work extends beyond the book. She has published narrative nonfiction essays in prestigious journals including The Examined Life Journal, Intima, CHEST (where she edits the narrative medicine section), and The New England

Journal of Medicine. Her essay "A View from the Edge: Creating a Culture of Caring" was published in NEJM and has been widely cited in discussions about healthcare culture change. She has written editorials for The Harvard Business Review, Annals of Internal Medicine, The Washington Post, and The Detroit Free Press, using her platform to advocate for systemic changes in how healthcare is delivered [1, 4].

Her essay "The Shape of the Shore" was awarded a Sydney by The New York Times and was nominated for a Pushcart Prize. In 2020, during the COVID-19 pandemic, the podcast This American Life documented the pandemic in Detroit in an episode titled "The Reprieve," using Dr. Awdish's audio diary of Henry Ford Hospital employees' experiences during that time. Her willingness to be vulnerable, to share her own struggles and fears, provided a powerful window into what healthcare workers were experiencing during one of the most challenging periods in modern medicine [1, 4].

Dr. Awdish has received numerous awards for her work. In 2016, she was named Critical Care Teacher of the Year by Henry Ford Health System [1, 4]. In 2017, she received the Schwartz Center's National Compassionate Caregiver of the Year Award and was named Physician of the Year by Press Ganey for her work on improving communication [1, 4]. She was inducted into the Gold Humanism Honor Society in 2019 and received the Ake Grenvik Honorary Award from the Society for Critical Care Medicine, one of the field's highest honors [2].

She has also been named a U.S. News Hospital Hero for her work on the front lines of the COVID-19 pandemic, where she treated her first infected patient on March 14, 2020 [2, 3, 10]. Throughout the pandemic, she continued to advocate for physician wellness and patient-centered care even as the system strained under unprecedented pressure.

Dr. Awdish is currently working on her second book, "After Shock," which is scheduled to be published by Macmillan in June 2026. The book has been described as "a piercingly honest, insightful, deeply vulnerable examination of the true nature of healing." Where "In Shock" was about the immediate experience of critical illness and the realization of medicine's failures, "After Shock" appears to be about the longer journey of healing; not just physical recovery but the deeper work of integrating trauma, finding meaning, and rebuilding a life after everything you believed has been shattered [11].

In interviews about the upcoming book, Dr. Awdish has spoken about healing as a "recursive process rather than a linear journey," one that requires "uncovering deeper layers of growth and emphasizing the power of listening, connection, and embodiment [12]." Seven years after writing "In Shock," she describes that first book as her "first pass" at understanding what happened to her. The second book represents a more mature, more nuanced exploration of what it means to truly heal, to not just survive but to thrive after catastrophic illness [1, 12].

Throughout her career since her illness, Dr. Awdish has continued to practice as a pulmonary and critical care physician at Henry Ford Hospital, where she serves as Director of the Pulmonary Hypertension Program [1, 2]. She maintains her clinical practice because, as she has explained, being with patients is essential to her understanding of medicine and healing. Her patients speak of her with profound gratitude, describing her as someone who truly sees them, who listens without rushing, who is willing to be fully present even in the most difficult moments [1].

Dr. Awdish is also a sought-after speaker who delivers keynote addresses to audiences ranging from professional medical societies to members of Congress to organizations combating homelessness [1, 13]. Her talks often focus on themes like "The Wound is the Gift," exploring how confronting mortality can help us find meaning and peace, and "The Broken Vessel," which examines what is needed to heal medicine itself. She speaks about the importance of giving primacy to the patient narrative, building resilience in physicians, and forming communities of care that can heal both patients and providers.

In addition to her clinical practice, her writing, and her speaking, Dr. Awdish maintains an active presence on social media, particularly the social network formerly named, Twitter, where she shares reflections on medicine, patient care, and the art her children create [14]. She also shares her own artwork, revealing another aspect of her creative life. Her social media presence is characterized by vulnerability, honesty, and a willingness to engage with difficult questions about medicine and healthcare.

As I read "In Shock" shortly after my own hospitalization, I found myself nodding along to so much of what Dr. Awdish described. The loss of agency that happens the moment you become a patient, even when you're a physician who should know better. The vulnerability of being in a hospital gown, of having your body exposed and examined, of having decisions made about you without adequate explanation or inclusion. The fear that comes from understanding enough medicine to know how bad things could get but not enough about your specific situation to know whether they will. The exhaustion of being woken throughout the night for vital signs and medications, of never being allowed to just rest and heal. The fishbowl experience of the ICU, where privacy is sacrificed to necessity but where that loss of privacy becomes another layer of indignity. But Dr. Awdish's book offered something more than validation of my experience. It offered a framework for understanding what had happened and what medicine could become. She demonstrated through her own transformation that physicians can learn to be present with suffering without being destroyed by it.

As I think about Dr. Rana Awdish's place among the physician-authors who have shaped modern medicine, I'm struck by how her contribution is both intensely personal and profoundly universal. The physician who nearly died has become the physician who teaches us all how to truly live; how to be present with suffering, how to maintain hope in the face of devastating illness, how to build genuine connections that heal both patients and physicians. The doctor who lost her unborn child and nearly lost her own life has become the doctor who helps all of us see that every life is precious, that every patient deserves to be seen as a whole person, that the work of medicine is ultimately about honoring the humanity in both ourselves and those we serve.

References

1. Awdish R. About. Rana Awdish MD. n.d. https://www.ranaawdishmd.com/about-5.
2. Henry Ford Health. Rana Awdish, MD. n.d. https://www.henryford.com/physician-directory/a/awdish-rana.
3. Wayne State University School of Medicine. U.S. News names physician and educator Rana Awdish, M.D. '02, a Hospital Hero. 2020, July 29. https://today.wayne.edu/medicine/news/2020/07/29/us-news-names-physician-and-educator-rana-awdish-md-02-a-hospital-hero-38698.
4. AAE Speakers. Rana Awdish keynote speaker. n.d. https://www.aaespeakers.com/keynote-speakers/rana-awdish.
5. American Medical Women's Association. AMWA member spotlight—Rana Awdish, MD. 2024, September 27. https://amwa-doc.org/amwa-member-spotlight-rana-awdish-md/.
6. Awdish R. In shock: my journey from death to recovery and the redemptive power of hope. New York: St. Martin's Press; 2017.
7. The Schwartz Center for Compassionate Healthcare. Rana Awdish, MD. 2017. https://www.theschwartzcenter.org/finalists/rana-awdish-md/.
8. Awdish R. A view from the edge—creating a culture of caring. N Engl J Med. 2017;376(1):7–9. https://doi.org/10.1056/NEJMp1614078.
9. Dayton K. (Host). Episode 116: "In Shock" with Dr. Rana Awdish [Audio podcast episode]. In Walking Home from the ICU. Dayton ICU Consulting; 2023, January 18. https://daytonicuconsulting.com/walking-home-from-the-icu-podcast/walking-home-from-the-icu-episode-episode-116-in-shock-with-dr-rana-awdish/.
10. U.S. News & World Report. Meet Rana Awdish, a critical care doctor on the coronavirus front lines. 2020, April 30. https://health.usnews.com/hospital-heroes/articles/meet-rana-awdish-a-critical-care-doctor-on-the-coronavirus-front-lines.
11. Awdish R. After shock. Macmillan; 2026. https://us.macmillan.com/books/9781250345837/aftershock/.
12. Silverman, E. (Host). The second pass at healing with Rana Awdish, MD [Audio podcast episode]. In The Nocturnists. 2024, December 12. https://thenocturnists.org/podcast/the-second-pass-at-healing-with-rana-awdish-md.
13. Macmillan Speakers Bureau. Rana Awdish, MD. n.d. https://www.macmillanspeakers.com/ranaawdish/.
14. Awdish R. [@RanaAwdish]. Tweets [X profile] X. n.d. https://x.com/RanaAwdish.

Chapter 7
Mona Hanna-Attisha, MD

Of all the Personal Statements I have written, the one I remain most proud of was for my residency application. I wrote, at the very end, that, "I yearn for a training that encourages, even compels me to grow in compassion and curiosity, that celebrates diversity and inspires inclusion, that is driven by innovation and fosters collegiality, that never shies away from the challenge of a patient who communicates differently; that cannot wait to one day solve the mystery, and that never stops looking for the clues." I envisioned myself in a deerstalker hat and cape, magnifying glass in hand as I tried to solve the mystery of the toddler who would not walk. Yet the mysteries of pediatrics extend outside the hospital and even beyond the clinic. Dr. Mona Hanna-Attisha solved one of those mysteries in Flint, Michigan, just north of where I completed my fellowship. Her work uncovered the pipeline of failed infrastructure and launched a movement to save thousands of children from lead poisoning.

Dr. Mona Hanna-Attisha was born on December 9, 1976, in Sheffield, England [1–3]. Her parents were Iraqi scientists and dissidents who had fled Saddam Hussein's repressive Ba'ath regime in the 1970s, seeking safety and freedom in a country where their scientific work and their political beliefs would not put them in mortal danger [4, 5]. They were Christians, members of a persecuted minority in Iraq, and they understood intimately what it meant to live under tyranny, to know that speaking truth could cost you everything [6].

Shortly after Mona was born, the family moved to the United States, eventually settling in Michigan [2]. They chose Flint initially, where Mona's mother taught English as a Second Language to other immigrants and her father, a metallurgical engineer, found work at General Motors [4, 6]. Later, the family moved to Royal Oak, a suburb of Detroit, where Mona would grow up straddling two worlds, the American dream her parents sought and the Iraqi heritage they carried with them, unable to return home for over 25 years [5]. Letters from grandparents arrived with sentences cut out by government censors. Family members disappeared or were tortured. The specter of authoritarianism, of governments that lie to their people and

O. M. Cox, *The Pen, The Stethoscope, and The Scalpel*,
https://doi.org/10.1007/978-3-032-19406-0_7

punish those who speak truth, was not an abstract concept in the Hanna household. It was lived experience, passed down through stories and silences, shaping Mona's understanding of what power could do and what resistance required [6].

This family history of activism and resistance would prove to be formative. While still a student at Kimball High School in Royal Oak, Mona became president of her class and joined a student environmental group [5]. When she learned that a polluting incinerator in a neighboring town was harming the community, she mobilized her classmates to help shut it down [7, 8]. The campaign succeeded. It was Mona's first taste of activism, her first experience of community organizing, her first proof that ordinary people—even teenagers—could challenge powerful interests and win. It was also where she met Elin Betanzo, a fellow member of the environmental club who would, years later, provide the tip that would change both their lives and the fate of Flint [7].

"Mona has always been an activist," Betanzo would later say. "She's always been willing to take a stand, especially for environmental causes [7]."

That early activism cemented Mona's commitment to environmental health and social justice. She went to the University of Michigan in Ann Arbor, where she earned a Bachelor of Science degree from the School for Environment and Sustainability [1, 7]. The program gave her a deep understanding of how environmental factors affect human health, how policy decisions cascade into real-world consequences, how the places we live determine our opportunities and our outcomes. It clearly encouraged her to think systemically; to see the connections between water quality and childhood development, between zoning laws and asthma rates, between poverty and de-prioritization.

But understanding environmental health wasn't enough. Mona wanted to be able to intervene directly, to care for the children most affected by environmental injustice. She applied to medical school, earning her Doctor of Medicine degree from Michigan State University College of Human Medicine in 2002 [1, 9]. At Michigan State, she was inducted into the Alpha Omega Alpha national medical honor society, a recognition of her academic excellence and her potential as a physician-leader [9].

Knowing that she would need more than clinical skills to address the root causes of illness, Mona also pursued a Master of Public Health degree in Health Management and Policy from the University of Michigan School of Public Health, which she completed in 2008 [1, 9]. The public health degree was crucial; it taught her epidemiology, biostatistics, health systems management, and most importantly, how to think about health problems at the population level. It gave her the methodological tools to conduct rigorous research and the credibility to defend that research when it was challenged. As one of her professors would later note, "It really made me feel good that she had the appropriate credentials to make her results valid [7]."

After completing medical school, Dr. Hanna-Attisha moved to New York City for her residency in pediatrics at Wayne State University/Children's Hospital of Michigan, where she also served as chief resident [10]. She fell in love with pediatrics; with the resilience of children, with the privilege of caring for them at their most vulnerable, with the opportunity to shape their futures through advocacy and care. She chose to specialize further, but not in a procedural subspecialty. Instead, she chose pediatric public health, a path that would allow her to combine clinical medicine with population-level interventions, to see individual patients while also working to change the systems that made them sick in the first place [3].

In 2011, Dr. Hanna-Attisha returned to Flint to become Director of the Pediatric Residency Program at Hurley Medical Center, a public hospital that served the city's most vulnerable residents [3, 10]. She also joined the faculty at Michigan State University College of Human Medicine. She had been in Flint briefly as a medical student, but this return was different. She was coming home not just to practice medicine but to train the next generation of physicians, to teach them how to care for children in one of America's most economically devastated cities.

Flint, once a thriving automotive manufacturing hub powered by General Motors, had been in decline for decades [11]. The auto industry had largely abandoned the city, taking with it the middle-class jobs that had sustained generations of families. Systemic racism had concentrated poverty and segregation. By 2011, nearly 70% of Flint's children under age five lived in poverty. The city's population had dropped from a high of nearly 200,000 to under 100,000 [11, 12]. Flint was, in many ways, a symbol of post-industrial urban America; a city left behind, struggling with crumbling infrastructure, insufficient tax base, and deep racial and economic inequality [13].

In 2011, Michigan's state government, dominated by Tea Party Republicans focused on austerity, declared Flint to be in a state of fiscal emergency. Rather than providing resources to help the city recover, the state effectively stripped Flint of its democracy, replacing the elected local government with a state-appointed emergency manager whose sole mandate was to cut costs. As Dr. Hanna-Attisha would later observe, it was no accident that the cities placed under emergency management were disproportionately Black. Flint, along with other predominantly African American communities, was "effectively colonized by the state [13]."

In April 2014, under the direction of the emergency manager, the city made a fateful decision: to save money, Flint would stop purchasing water from Detroit, which drew from Lake Huron and the Great Lakes system. Instead, Flint would begin drawing its water from the Flint River, a waterway that had been used for decades as an industrial dumping ground [14]. The switch would save approximately $5 million over 2 years.

Residents immediately noticed problems. The water looked brown, smelled strange, tasted metallic. People developed rashes. Some reported hair loss. Residents complained, but they were told the water was safe. Tests showed elevated bacteria levels, leading to boil water advisories, but officials insisted that once the bacteria issue was resolved, the water was fine. General Motors stopped using Flint water in its engine plant because it was corroding machine parts, but residents were assured it was safe for them to drink, to bathe in, to use for cooking and making baby formula [7].

Dr. Hanna-Attisha, like most Flint residents, was concerned but reassured by official statements. "Flint was literally in the middle of the Great Lakes region, the largest source of freshwater in the world," she would later write. "Why doubt the safety of what was coming out of the tap? [15]" She trusted that the people whose job it was to protect public health were doing exactly that. As a pediatrician, she told worried parents—including parents who directly asked her about the water—that it was safe.

And then came the barbecue that changed everything.

In August 2015, Dr. Hanna-Attisha's old high school friend Elin Betanzo, now a water systems consultant who had previously worked at the EPA during the Washington D.C. water crisis, came to visit [7, 11]. Over wine and conversation, Betanzo mentioned that the Flint water wasn't being treated properly. The city, in its cost-cutting measures, had not added corrosion control chemicals to the water treatment process [11, 14]. Corrosion control is standard practice, especially with water as corrosive as the Flint River, because without it, the water leaches lead from old pipes. And much of Flint's water infrastructure was built with lead pipes.

"When I heard about lead," Dr. Hanna-Attisha later said, "my life changed [11]."

As a pediatrician, she knew exactly what lead exposure meant for children. Lead is a neurotoxin with no safe level of exposure. It causes irreversible brain damage, developmental delays, decreased IQ, memory and attention problems, learning disabilities, speech issues, and increased risk for aggressive behavior and serious chronic conditions [11, 14]. Lead poisoning doesn't just affect one child's life; it affects their entire trajectory, their ability to learn, to work, to thrive. And because the effects are irreversible, exposure in early childhood creates deficits that persist for a lifetime.

Dr. Hanna-Attisha was horrified. She immediately thought of her patients; the children she saw in clinic, the children whose growth and development she monitored, the children whose parents trusted her to keep them safe. If the water was contaminated with lead, those children were being poisoned. Every day, with every glass of water, every bath, every meal prepared with Flint water, they were accumulating lead in their bodies and brains [11, 15].

She knew she had to act. But she also knew that accusations without evidence would be dismissed. She needed data. She needed proof. She needed science that was so rigorous, so irrefutable, that officials would have no choice but to acknowledge the truth.

"I knew that if I was going to make a difference, I would need science, data and facts in my pocket," she later explained [11].

Working quickly, Dr. Hanna-Attisha launched a study using Hurley Medical Center's electronic medical records [3, 14]. She and her team analyzed the blood lead levels of children under 5 years old in Flint, comparing the levels before and after the April 2014 water switch. The analysis was straightforward but damning: the percentage of Flint children with elevated blood lead levels had nearly doubled since the city started drawing water from the Flint River. In some neighborhoods, the numbers had nearly tripled [7, 14].

She verified her methodology, checked her statistics, confirmed her results. There was no question: Flint's children were being poisoned by their drinking water.

Now came the hard part: going public.

On September 24, 2015, Dr. Hanna-Attisha did something most doctors never have to do. She walked out of her clinic wearing her white coat and stood up in one of Hurley Medical Center's hospital conference rooms, where residents typically attended lectures. There, she held a press conference, sharing her research findings and demanding immediate action to protect Flint's children [4, 11, 14].

The backlash was swift and brutal.

State officials didn't acknowledge the problem or thank her for bringing it to their attention. Instead, they attacked her. They accused her of "splicing and dicing" data, of using flawed methodology, of causing "near hysteria." A state spokesperson called her "an unfortunate researcher" and claimed her data set was different from the state's data. The Michigan Department of Environmental Quality spokesman acted, as she would later describe him, like "a rabid pit bull," dismissing her concerns and defending the state's position that the water was safe [11, 14].

Dr. Hanna-Attisha was blindsided. She had expected that presenting scientific evidence of harm to children would prompt immediate protective action. Instead, she was being publicly discredited by the very government agencies whose job it was to protect public health.

"I felt absolutely tiny and defeated," she recalled. "I began to second guess myself. I think, especially so many women, we often talk about imposter syndrome. I felt like I shouldn't have done this [11]."

But she did not back down. She rechecked her data. She verified her analysis again and again. She knew she was right. And she had allies: her hospital administration supported her, her family believed in her, and Virginia Tech professor Marc Edwards—the whistleblower who had exposed the Washington D.C. lead crisis—reached out to share his own research showing that Flint's tap water contained dangerous levels of lead [3].

Within days, the Detroit Free Press published its own analysis of the state's data, confirming that Dr. Hanna-Attisha's findings were accurate [4, 11]. Shortly after, the state's chief medical officer conceded that her analysis was sound. A federal emergency was declared. Lead filters and bottled water were distributed to Flint residents. Eventually, after officials had initially insisted it was impossible, the water source was switched back to Lake Huron [4].

Dr. Hanna-Attisha had been vindicated. But vindication was not what she wanted.

"I don't want to be vindicated," she said. "I just want the kids to be protected. Our kids never should have had to go through this. I'm glad that we were able to expose all this, but it never should've happened in the first place [11]."

The damage, both to Flint's water infrastructure and to its children, had already been done. As many as 27,000 children had been exposed to elevated lead levels [7]. Thanks to Dr. Hanna-Attisha's efforts, Flint received over $350 million in state and federal aid [16]. But she was determined that Flint's response to the crisis would also last a lifetime.

In 2016, she founded the Michigan State University and Hurley Children's Hospital Pediatric Public Health Initiative, dedicated to mitigating the impact of lead exposure on Flint's children [9]. The program takes a comprehensive, proactive approach, recognizing that while there is no medication to reverse lead poisoning, there are evidence-based interventions that can promote brain development and limit the crisis's long-term impact. The initiative provides universal developmental screening, nutritional support including a fruit and vegetable prescription program, early childhood education, home visiting programs, and wraparound services for families [9].

"We cannot ethically wait to see the consequences of lead poisoning," Dr. Hanna-Attisha explained. "We can't take away lead. I wish I could prescribe a magic pill or an antidote to take away lead poisoning; there is no such thing. But we can do a lot to limit children's exposure to mitigate the impact of this crisis [17]."

The work was personal for Dr. Hanna-Attisha, who had her own two young daughters at home. At the height of the crisis, she was hardly ever with them. They understood, she would later say, that their mother was with their 6000 siblings [11].

Dr. Hanna-Attisha testified multiple times before the United States Congress, calling for federal action to replace lead pipes and strengthen regulations around lead in drinking water [9]. Her advocacy helped push the EPA to propose, in 2024, the first major revisions to 30-year-old lead-in-water regulations, including requirements to replace lead service lines within a decade, enhanced testing requirements, and lowering the action level for lead from 15 parts per billion to 10 parts per billion [4, 9].

In 2018, Dr. Hanna-Attisha published her memoir, "What the Eyes Don't See: A Story of Crisis, Resistance, and Hope in an American City." The book, published by Penguin Random House's One World imprint, tells the story of the Flint water crisis through Dr. Hanna-Attisha's eyes, both as a physician caring for poisoned children and as the daughter of Iraqi immigrants whose family history of resistance prepared her to stand up to power [15].

The title comes from a slightly altered D.H. Lawrence quote: "The eyes don't see what the mind doesn't know." It speaks to how Dr. Hanna-Attisha and other Flint residents had been drinking contaminated water without recognizing the danger, how officials ignored evidence they didn't want to acknowledge, how systemic problems become invisible when we trust that someone else is taking care of them.

The book is paced like a scientific thriller, moving between Dr. Hanna-Attisha's personal story—her family's journey from Saddam Hussein's Iraq to suburban Michigan, her path to medicine and public health, her growth as an activist—and the urgent detective work of uncovering the water crisis [15]. She writes with moral outrage tempered by hope, refusing to let Flint be defined solely by this crisis while also insisting that what happened in Flint was not an isolated incident but a symptom of deeper national problems: environmental injustice, structural racism, deteriorating infrastructure, disrespect for science, and a failure to care for our most vulnerable citizens [13].

"What the Eyes Don't See" became a New York Times Notable Book and received widespread critical acclaim. The New York Times Book Review called it "gripping... entertaining... Her book has power precisely because she takes the events she recounts so personally... Moral outrage present on every page." The Washington Post described it as "a clarion call to live a life of purpose." O: The Oprah Magazine compared it to "a Grisham thriller." Erin Brockovich, the famous environmental activist, called Dr. Hanna-Attisha "a true American hero" [1, 3].

The book has been widely adopted in medical school curricula and university courses on public health, environmental justice, and urban policy. It provides not just an account of the Flint water crisis but a case study in how systemic failures compound, how racism and austerity politics create conditions for disaster, and how ordinary people can resist even when the odds seem impossible [1, 9].

For her role in exposing the Flint water crisis and her ongoing advocacy, Dr. Hanna-Attisha has received numerous honors. In 2016, Time magazine named her one of the 100 Most Influential People in the World. She was included in Politico's Politico 50, named Michiganian of the Year by the Detroit News, and selected as one of the Ten Outstanding Young Americans. She received the 2016 Ridenhour Prize for Truth-Telling and the PEN American Center's James C. Goodale Freedom of Expression Courage Award [9, 15, 18, 19]. She was awarded the Rose Nader Award for Arab American activism by the American-Arab Anti-Discrimination Committee and named Champion of Justice by ACCESS (Arab Community Center for Economic and Social Services) [4].

In 2022, she received the inaugural Bernard Lown Award for Social Responsibility from the Lown Institute, which came with a $25,000 prize that she donated to the Flint Kids Fund [20]. U.S. News named her a Hospital Hero for her work on the front lines of the COVID-19 pandemic in Detroit. She was inducted into the Gold Humanism Honor Society and has been named Compassionate Caregiver of the Year [10, 15, 21].

Dr. Hanna-Attisha has become a sought-after speaker, delivering keynote addresses to audiences ranging from medical conferences to congressional hearings to universities to organizations combating homelessness. She speaks about environmental justice, the power of speaking truth to power, the importance of listening to communities, and the responsibility physicians have to advocate for systemic change. In 2016, she was the commencement speaker at Michigan State University, Johns Hopkins School of Public Health, Virginia Tech, and numerous other institutions [4, 22].

Dr. Hanna Attisha continues to practice pediatrics and serves as Associate Dean and Professor of Public Health at Michigan State University College of Human Medicine. She trains the next generation of physicians and public health practitioners, teaching them not just clinical skills but also the courage to speak up when they see injustice, the humility to listen to patients and communities, and the persistence to fight for change even when powerful interests resist.

Her work extends beyond Flint. She has become an international champion for safe water and a fierce spokesperson for children in poverty everywhere. She advocates for infrastructure investment, for strengthening environmental regulations, for dismantling the structural racism that allows some communities to be poisoned while others are protected. She calls for what she describes as a fundamental principle: "It's about not being OK with poisoned water, and it's about not being OK with babies growing up in poverty [23]."

As Flint commemorates the tenth anniversary of its water crisis, Dr. Hanna-Attisha emphasizes that the crisis does not define the city. "Flint will not be defined by this crisis," she insists. Instead, Flint will be defined by how its community came together; how residents organized, how activists persisted, how physicians like her used their platforms to amplify community voices, how parents fought for their children, how the city refused to accept that children born in Flint deserved any less than children born anywhere else.

The story of Flint is, in Dr. Hanna-Attisha's telling, ultimately a story of resistance, activism, and hope. It is about what becomes possible when people refuse to accept injustice, when they insist on being heard, when they use whatever tools they have—whether medical records, statistical analysis, press conferences, or grassroots organizing—to fight for what is right.

Her story reminds me why I wrote what I did in my residency personal statement about solving mysteries. The toddler who won't walk might have a neuromuscular disease, or developmental delay, or a metabolic disorder. Those are the mysteries we train to solve in the hospital. But Dr. Hanna-Attisha solved a different sort of mystery: Why were Flint's children getting sick? The answer wasn't a rare genetic syndrome or an exotic infection. The answer was environmental racism, government negligence, and infrastructure failure. The answer was that powerful people had decided that saving money could be achieved at the expense of protecting children.

The mysteries I wanted to solve when I wrote my residency personal statement—the diagnostic puzzles, the unusual presentations, the rare syndromes—remain important. But Dr. Hanna-Attisha has underscored the larger mysteries which plague communities around the country. Why do some children have more exposure to lead than others? Why do asthma rates vary so dramatically by neighborhood? Why do infant mortality rates remain so much higher for Black babies than white babies? Why are some communities' voices heard while others are ignored?

These are mysteries that require not just clinical acumen but also epidemiological analysis, historical understanding, political engagement, and moral courage. They are mysteries that cannot be solved by individual physicians working alone, but they cannot be solved without physicians willing to use their expertise and their platform to fight for change.

Dr. Mona Hanna-Attisha has given us a blueprint for how to be that kind of physician. She has shown us that a white coat can be a tool for activism, that a medical degree carries responsibilities that extend far beyond the exam room, that the oath to protect patients sometimes requires us to challenge the very authorities we were taught to trust.

References

1. Hanna-Attisha M. About. Dr. Mona. n.d. https://monahannaattisha.com/about.
2. Mason J. Pathbreakers of Arab America—Mona Hanna, MD. Arab America. 2025, October 8. https://www.arabamerica.com/pathbreakers-of-arab-america-mona-hanna-md/.
3. Yale Environmental Professionals of Color. Hanna-Attisha, Mona. Justice, Equity, Diversity, and Sustainability Initiative. n.d. https://environmental-professionals-of-color.yale.edu/person/hanna-attisha-mona.

4. Americans Who Tell The Truth. Dr. Mona Hanna. n.d. https://americanswhotellthetruth.org/portraits/dr-mona-hanna-attisha/.
5. American University of Beirut. Mona Hanna-Attisha. Honorary Doctorates. n.d. https://aub.edu.lb/doctorates/recipients/Pages/Mona_Hanna.aspx.
6. American Immigration Council. Iraqi-American doctor who blew whistle on Flint water crisis asks, what if I hadn't been here? 2017, February 23. https://www.newamericaneconomy.org/feature/iraqi-american-doctor-who-blew-whistle-on-flint-water-crisis-asks-what-if-i-hadnt-been-here/.
7. University of Michigan Alumni Association. The hero of Flint's water crisis. n.d. https://alumni.umich.edu/michigan-alum/the-hero-of-flints-water-crisis/.
8. Crain's Detroit Business. Mona Hanna-Attisha—2021 most influential women. 2021, November 8. https://www.crainsdetroit.com/awards/mona-hanna-attisha-2021-most-influential-women.
9. Michigan State University College of Human Medicine. Mona Hanna, MD, MPH, FAAP. n.d. https://humanmedicine.msu.edu/directory/hanna-mona.html.
10. Hurley Medical Education & Research. Mona Hanna. n.d. https://education.hurleymc.com/people/mona-hanna/.
11. NIH Record. Pediatrician who uncovered Flint water crisis recounts experience. 2021, April 30. https://nihrecord.nih.gov/2021/04/30/pediatrician-who-uncovered-flint-water-crisis-recounts-experience.
12. PBS NewsHour. A new program 'prescribes' monthly payments for the first year of an infant's life. 2024, February 19. https://www.pbs.org/newshour/health/a-new-anti-poverty-program-in-flint-michigan-gives-cash-to-new-moms.
13. Kirkus Reviews. What the eyes don't see. n.d. https://www.kirkusreviews.com/book-reviews/mona-hanna-attisha/what-the-eyes-dont-see/.
14. PEN America. 2016 PEN/Toni and James C. Goodale Freedom of Expression Courage Award: Lee-Anne Walters and Dr. Mona Hanna-Attisha. 2016. https://pen.org/2016-pentoni-and-james-c-goodale-freedom-of-expression-courage-award-lee-anne-walters-and-dr-mona-hanna-attisha/.
15. Hanna Attisha M. What the eyes don't see: a story of crisis, resistance, and hope in an American city. One World/Random House; 2018. https://www.penguinrandomhouse.com/books/550935/what-the-eyes-dont-see-by-mona-hanna-attisha/.
16. S.A.F.E. For Children. Spotlight of the week: Dr. Mona Hanna-Attisha—the pediatrician who refused to look away. 2025, June 2. https://childreninfobank.com/spotlight-of-the-week-dr-mona-hanna-attisha-the-pediatrician-who-refused-to-look-away/.
17. Gross T. Pediatrician who exposed Flint water crisis shares her "story of resistance." NPR. 2018, June 25. https://www.npr.org/sections/health-shots/2018/06/25/623126968/pediatrician-who-exposed-flint-water-crisis-shares-her-story-of-resistance.
18. Carnegie Corporation of New York. Dr. Mona Hanna: Awards. n.d.. https://www.carnegie.org/awards/honoree/mona-hanna-attisha/.
19. Michigan State University. Mona Hanna-Attisha named one of TIME's most influential people. MSU Today. 2016, April 21. https://msutoday.msu.edu/news/2016/mona-hanna-attisha-named-one-of-times-most-influential-people.
20. Lown Institute. Pediatrician who uncovered Flint water crisis wins national award for social responsibility in medicine. 2022, June 6. https://lowninstitute.org/pediatrician-who-uncovered-flint-water-crisis-wins-national-award-for-social-responsibility-in-medicine%EF%BF%BC/.
21. Michigan State University Honored Faculty. Mona Hanna. n.d. https://msu.edu/honored-faculty/directory/attisha-hanna-mona.html.
22. Penguin Random House Speakers Bureau. Dr. Mona Hanna: Public health advocate. n.d. https://www.prhspeakers.com/speaker/dr-mona-hanna.
23. McCormick E. Michigan doctor who revealed Flint water crisis now takes on child poverty. The Guardian. 2024, April 25. https://www.theguardian.com/us-news/2024/apr/25/flint-michigan-child-poverty.

Chapter 8
Louise Aronson, MD

In my first year as an attending, I approached the concept of Halloween with some mild trepidation and moderate excitement. I would be going into my clinic as a character from the Sims™. I had cardboard green plumbobs attached to headbands to allow the whole team to get in on the fun (should they choose). It was the sort of easy costume that could be taken off for serious conversations but might otherwise inject some humor into a child's otherwise hectic visit to the hospital. I revealed my hand-crafted costume to the team to gratifying wows, while I helpfully clarified that we might be all Sims characters. And then the first-year medical student asked me what the Sims was. At least five new grey hairs sprouted above my brow as I realized that what had once been a popular pastime for the kids had been edged aside by Roblox. Our brilliant medical student had also asked me who Zelda—the Princess—was, so I also considered that her interests just did not run on those tracks. Until my teenage patient referred to the game as one her grandmother played. I kept my plumbob, but also accepted that I was finally—happily—old. The experience of aging, and of seeing parents, children, loved ones, grow in time, is the fate of all of us, should we be so lucky. It is a journey fraught with inevitability, with entrance granted via a one-way ticket. The lessons we learn as the train ambles along are best sketched in the book, "Elderhood: Redefining Aging, Transforming Medicine, Reimagining Life." Dr. Louise Aronson uses brilliant watercolors to render a future we both expect and must accept. Her art is critical as is her continued work as a geriatrician, and I am pleased to share both with you.

Dr. Louise Aronson was born in 1963 in San Francisco, California, at the very medical center where she would one day work as a professor and practicing physician. She is a fifth-generation San Franciscan, a fact that sometimes leads her to joke that she hasn't gone very far in life, "just down 15 floors and over a building or two [1]." But this geographic continuity belies the remarkable journey she has taken from childhood dreamer to physician-writer, from someone who wanted to help people to someone who has transformed how we think about an entire stage of human life.

O. M. Cox, *The Pen, The Stethoscope, and The Scalpel*,
https://doi.org/10.1007/978-3-032-19406-0_8

As a child, Louise had two distinct aspirations that seemed, on the surface, contradictory. She wanted to become either the next Max Perkins—the legendary Scribner editor who worked with Hemingway and Fitzgerald—or a professional basketball player. The latter dream, she would later admit with humor, was "doomed from the start by her vertical, visual, and coordination challenges [1]." But the former dream, the love of stories and the desire to shape narratives that would move people and change minds, would prove to be foundational even as she took what seemed like a completely different path into medicine.

Louise attended college as a History and Anthropology major, drawn to understanding human societies and the stories of how people lived. She chose medicine, she has said, "in hopes of improving human lives," pursuing her undergraduate degree with the intellectual curiosity of someone who wanted to understand not just biological systems but human systems; how societies work, how cultures shape experience, how individual lives unfold within larger historical contexts [1].

She went to Harvard Medical School for her medical degree, immersing herself in the rigorous scientific training that would prepare her to diagnose disease and prescribe treatments. But even in medical school, Louise was already thinking about the stories behind the symptoms, the narrative arc of illness, the way that disease transforms not just bodies but lives. She completed her residency in Internal Medicine at the University of California, San Francisco, the institution where she had been born and where she would eventually make her career [2, 3].

After residency, Dr. Aronson pursued fellowship training in both clinical care and medical education. She became a geriatrician, specializing in the care of older adults [2]. It would be a choice that revealed her interests in the long arc of human life, in the complexity of aging bodies and minds, in the challenges of caring for people who have accumulated decades of experience and medical history [1].

But something was missing. Despite her success as a physician, despite finding fulfillment in caring for her patients, Dr. Aronson felt the pull of that childhood dream. She wanted to write. She wanted to tell stories. She wanted, as she would later discover, to be "at least as useful with a pen or keyboard as with a prescription pad and stethoscope [1]."

So, she did what seemed improbable: she went back to school. While working as a full-time physician, Dr. Aronson earned her Master of Fine Arts (MFA) in fiction writing from the Warren Wilson Program for Writers, one of the most prestigious low-residency MFA programs in the country [1, 3]. Warren Wilson is known for its rigorous curriculum, its emphasis on close reading and revision, and its commitment to developing writers who can craft stories with both artistry and meaning [4].

The MFA wasn't just a sideline or a hobby. It was Dr. Aronson reclaiming the part of herself that had always wanted to be: an editor, a writer, a storyteller. It was her recognition that the most important stories she encountered weren't in books but in her office. In 2013, Dr. Aronson published her first book, "A History of the Present Illness," a collection of short stories published by Bloomsbury [1, 5]. The title comes from medical terminology, the "history of the present illness" (HPI) is the critical first portion of the medical note that describes the onset, duration, character, context, and severity of illness. Basically, as Dr. Aronson explains, "it's the story, and without it, you can't understand what's going on with your patient [1]."

The collection takes readers into overlooked lives in the neighborhoods, hospitals, and nursing homes of San Francisco, offering what reviewers called "a deeply humane and incisive portrait of health and illness in America today [1]." The stories feature a remarkable range of voices: an elderly Chinese immigrant who sacrifices his demented wife's well-being to his son's authority; a busy Latina physician whose eldest daughter's need for attention has disastrous consequences; a young veteran whose injuries become a metaphor for the rest of his life; a gay doctor who learns very different lessons about family from his life and his work; a psychiatrist who advocates for the underserved but may herself be struggling with mental illness [1, 6].

Dr. Aronson wrote these stories in the tradition of physician-writers like William Carlos Williams and Anton Chekhov, but with her own distinctive voice; what critics described as "tender," "empathetic," and "unflinchingly honest." The New York Times praised her "lovely, nuanced description [1, 5]." The San Francisco Chronicle noted that the collection provides "an intimate look into how the aging process affects real lives and a non-didactic take on the importance of health care." The Independent (UK) observed that "the ethical dilemmas that abound in medicine are prominent but never swamp the stories: these are tales about people, as insightful as Lorrie Moore or Alice Munro [1, 5]."

The book earned Dr. Aronson significant literary recognition. She received a MacDowell fellowship, the prestigious residency program that provides artists with time and space to work. She won the Sonora Review Prize and received four Pushcart Prize nominations, a remarkable achievement given that the Pushcart Prize is one of the most respected honors in American literature for work published in small presses and literary journals [1].

"A History of the Present Illness" demonstrated that Dr. Aronson could write fiction that was both artistically accomplished and deeply informed by medical experience. She didn't write what are sometimes dismissively called "doctor stories," she wrote stories about human beings facing difficult situations, stories that happened to be illuminated by medical knowledge but were fundamentally about the human condition. The stories featured characters from diverse backgrounds and didn't offer easy answers to their problems. Instead, they offered a glimpse of the inevitable human battle with the vicissitudes of life.

But Dr. Aronson wasn't done. As accomplished as "A History of the Present Illness" was, she had something larger to say, not through fiction but through the kind of sweeping cultural analysis and personal reflection that only nonfiction could provide. She wanted to write about aging, about how we think about old age, about how medicine treats (and mistreats) older adults, about what it means to be human in the final decades of life.

In 2019, Dr. Aronson published "Elderhood: Redefining Aging, Transforming Medicine, Reimagining Life," also published by Bloomsbury [7]. The book was immediately recognized as something extraordinary; a work that combined memoir, cultural criticism, medical analysis, historical research, and visionary thinking into a comprehensive meditation on what it means to grow old in America [8].

"Elderhood" draws on Dr. Aronson's quarter century of experience caring for older patients, her observations of her own parents aging, and her research into history, science, literature, and popular culture. The book's central argument is both simple and revolutionary: we have made a catastrophic mistake by treating old age as a disease, as something to be dreaded, denigrated, neglected, and denied.

Dr. Aronson points out that for more than 5000 years, "old" has been defined as beginning between the ages of 60 and 70 [1]. That means most people alive today will spend more years in elderhood than in childhood, and many will be elders for 40 years or more. Yet at the very moment that humans are living longer than ever before, our culture has decided that aging is something to fight against rather than something to embrace as a distinct and valuable stage of life.

The book is structured around three sections corresponding to the three traditional stages of life—childhood, adulthood, and elderhood—but Dr. Aronson makes clear that these are cultural constructs, not biological inevitabilities. She examines how societies have understood aging across time and cultures, how medical education systematically neglects geriatrics (most medical students receive minimal training in caring for older adults despite the fact that the majority of their future patients will be elderly), how our healthcare system is designed around the needs and characteristics of middle-aged adults rather than the very different needs of older people, and how ageism permeates our culture in ways we barely recognize.

Throughout the book, Dr. Aronson weaves together patient stories, personal anecdotes (including her experiences caring for her aging parents), historical research, and sharp cultural analysis. She writes with what reviewers called "empathy," "wit," "moral outrage," and "hope [1, 7, 9]." She is candid about the challenges of aging; the losses, the indignities, the ways that bodies and minds change, the reality of approaching death. But she refuses to accept that these challenges make elderhood inherently miserable or worthless.

Instead, Dr. Aronson offers a vision of old age that is "neither nightmare nor utopian fantasy," a vision that acknowledges suffering while also recognizing joy, wonder, continued growth, wisdom, pleasure, purpose, and connection [1, 7]. She argues that we need to transform not just how medicine treats older people but how our entire culture thinks about aging. We need better training for healthcare providers, better systems of care, better public policies, and most fundamentally, a cultural shift that allows us to see elderhood not as decline but as a distinct life stage with its own developmental tasks, opportunities, and values.

"Elderhood" was published to extraordinary acclaim. It became a New York Times Bestseller. It was named a finalist for the 2020 Pulitzer Prize for General Nonfiction, one of the highest honors in American letters. It was longlisted for the Andrew Carnegie Medal for Excellence in Nonfiction. It won the WSU AOS Bonner Book Award and the 2022 At Home With Growing Older Impact Award [1, 2].

Critics compared it to Atul Gawande's "Being Mortal" and Oliver Sacks's work [7]. Kirkus Reviews, gave it a starred review, described it as "empathetic, probing, and often emotionally moving narratives on appreciating the power and the pain of aging [9]." Dr. Lucy Kalanithi, whose work, "When Breath Becomes Air" (completed after her husband Paul's death) had become a phenomenon, praised "Elderhood" effusively: "As Louise Aronson says, 'Life offers just two possibilities: die young or grow old.' This searing, luminous book is for everyone who hopes to accomplish the latter and remain fully human as they do. It will challenge your assumptions and open your mind—and it just might change your life [7]."

Dr. Perri Klass wrote: "In Elderhood, Louise Aronson draws on the experiences of her own life and the many lives she has touched as a geriatrician to think about age and aging, combining the insights of science and medicine with the wisdom of literature and human history, all narrated with the practical realism of the caring clinician. It's a wise and beautiful book, to be cherished by anyone who hopes to keep on growing, aging, and learning [7]."

Dr. Abraham Verghese, author of "Cutting for Stone" and himself a master of medical narrative, said: "In the latter years there are possibilities for joy, transcendence, and meaning, but also for just the opposite. Aronson writes like a memoirist while giving us scientific insight, philosophical wisdom, and wise counsel for a journey and destination we all share. Elderhood is a lovely and thoughtful exploration of this voyage [7]."

The book appeared on countless "best of" lists and became required or recommended reading not just in medical schools but in schools of public health, nursing programs, social work programs, and courses on aging, health policy, and cultural studies [1]. It reached far beyond the medical community to general readers who were confronting their own aging or caring for aging parents, who were worried about growing old in a society that doesn't value older people, who wanted a different vision of what the last decades of life could be.

Dr. Aronson has said that she wrote "Elderhood" because "the most important stories, and the ones that made my work so meaningful and fulfilling, were the ones I heard in my office: the stories of real people of all ages and backgrounds [1]." She wanted to share those stories, to use them to illuminate larger truths about aging, medicine, and what it means to be human.

Beyond her books, Dr. Aronson has published extensively in both medical and literary venues. Her articles and essays have appeared in The New York Times, The Washington Post, Discover Magazine, The New England Journal of Medicine, The Lancet, Health Affairs, JAMA, Annals of Internal Medicine, the Journal of the American Geriatrics Society, Bellevue Literary Review, and Narrative Magazine [1, 10, 11]. She writes with equal facility for medical audiences and general readers, translating complex medical concepts for lay readers and bringing literary sensibility to medical discourse. Her work has been featured on Today, CBS This Morning, NPR's Fresh Air, Politico, LitHub, Kaiser Health News, and Tech Nation [3, 10]. She has become a sought-after speaker and commentator on aging, medical education, and the intersection of medicine and humanities.

Throughout her writing career, Dr. Aronson has continued to practice medicine and teach. She is a Professor of Medicine at UCSF, where she has held numerous leadership roles [2, 3]. She has served as director of the Northern California Geriatrics Education Center, the UCSF Pathways to Discovery program, and the

Optimizing Aging Project. She was Chief of Geriatrics Education and currently leads the campus-wide Health Humanities and Social Advocacy Initiative. She founded the Optimizing Aging practice at the UCSF Osher Center for Integrative Health, where she continues to care for older adults [1–3].

Her work as a medical educator has been recognized with numerous awards. She received the Arnold P. Gold Foundation Professorship for her project "Fostering Humanism through Critical Reflection and Narrative Advocacy [2, 3]." She was awarded the UCSF Medical Education Research Fellowship and the 2011 Cooke Award for the Scholarship of Teaching and Learning [8]. From 2010 to 2016, she was a member of UCSF's Academy of Medical Educators. She has received the American Geriatrics Society's Outstanding Mid-Career Clinician Educator of the Year Award (also known as the Clinician-Teacher of the Year Award), the California Homecare Physician of the Year Award, and was inducted into the Gold Humanism Honor Society [1–3, 8].

Dr. Aronson's research has focused on geriatrics education, reflective learning in medicine (which emphasizes learning from experience to improve care), health advocacy, and medical writing for the public. She has developed innovative curricula for teaching medical students and residents about aging, about communicating with older patients and their families, about the social determinants of health that shape aging experiences, and about how to practice medicine with humanism and cultural humility [3].

One of Dr. Aronson's signature contributions to medical education is her work on reflective learning. She developed "The UCSF LEaP: A Guide for Reflective Learning in Medical Education," published in MedEdPORTAL, which provides a framework for helping medical learners reflect on their experiences and develop greater insight into their own practice [2]. She also created "The UCSF Faculty Development Workshop on Critical Reflection in Medical Education," training educators to teach and provide feedback on learners' reflections [2].

She has been named one of Next Avenue's 2019 Influencers in Aging and received the 2019-2020 Humanism in Aging Leadership Award, as well as the American Geriatrics Society's Outstanding Mid-Career Clinician Educator of the Year Award [12, 13]. These honors recognize not just her clinical excellence or her literary achievements but her role in changing how we think about and care for older adults.

Dr. Aronson teaches us that the same developmental tasks that challenge children and adolescents also challenge older adults: figuring out who you are, finding purpose and meaning, maintaining relationships, adapting to change, learning new skills, contributing to your community. The tasks don't end at 60 or 70. They continue, taking different forms but remaining essential to human flourishing.

She also teaches us that medicine has failed older adults in systematic ways. Medical training focuses overwhelmingly on acute illness in younger and middle-aged adults. Doctors learn to diagnose rare diseases but not how to manage the complex interplay of multiple chronic conditions that characterize aging. Hospitals are designed for efficiency and cure rather than for the comfort and dignity of older patients who may need more time, more explanation, and more attention to the social and emotional aspects of care. Clinical trials exclude older adults, meaning we have limited evidence about how medications work in the very population most likely to need them.

Finally, Dr. Aronson teaches us that these failures are not inevitable. We can train doctors differently. We can design care systems differently. We can develop medications specifically for older adults. We can change how hospitals work, how nursing homes operate, how communities support aging residents. We can create a culture that values the contributions of older adults, that sees the last decades of life as a time of continued growth and purpose rather than just decline and loss.

As I grow older—as I accumulate more grey hairs, as my cultural references become more dated, as I move closer to elderhood myself—I find great comfort in Dr. Louise Aronson's vision. She is a reminder that aging is not a disease to be cured but a stage of life to be lived. That the challenges of aging are real, but so are the opportunities. That there is joy to be found, wisdom to be gained, purpose to be pursued, connections to be deepened, even in the final decades of life.

References

1. Aronson L. About. Louise Aronson. n.d. https://louisearonson.com/about/.
2. UCSF Profiles. Louise Aronson, MD MFA. n.d. https://profiles.ucsf.edu/louise.aronson.
3. UCSF Health. Louise Aronson, MD, MFA. n.d. https://www.ucsfhealth.org/providers/dr-louise-aronson.
4. 14 Hills & Williams M. Louise Aronson [Interview]. n.d. https://www.14hills.net/interview-louise-aronson.
5. Aronson L. A history of the present illness. Bloomsbury Publishing; 2013. https://louisearonson.com/books/a-history-of-the-present-illness/.
6. GeriPal Podcast. "A History of the Present Illness," a new book by Dr. Louise Aronson. 2013, February. https://geripal.org/a-history-of-present-illness-new-book/.
7. Aronson L. Elderhood: redefining aging, transforming medicine, reimagining life. Bloomsbury Publishing; 2019. https://louisearonson.com/books/elderhood/.
8. UCSF Division of Geriatrics. Louise Aronson publish new book: 'Elderhood.' 2019. https://geriatrics.ucsf.edu/news/louise-aronson-publish-new-book-elderhood-redefining-aging-transforming-medicine-reimagining.
9. Kirkus Reviews. Elderhood. 2019. https://www.kirkusreviews.com/book-reviews/louise-aronson/elderhood/.
10. UCSF Department of Humanities and Social Sciences. Louise Aronson, MD, MFA. n.d. https://humsci.ucsf.edu/people/louise-aronson-md-mfa.
11. Narrative Magazine. Louise Aronson. n.d. https://www.narrativemagazine.com/authors/louise-aronson.
12. NY Writers Institute. Coronavirus and compassion: Dr. Louise Aronson is looking out for older Americans. 2020, May 5 https://www.nyswritersinstitute.org/post/coronavirus-and-compassion-dr-louise-aronson-is-looking-out-for-older-americans.
13. American Geriatrics Society. Outstanding Mid-career clinician educator of the year award. n.d. https://www.americangeriatrics.org/about-us/awards/outstanding-mid-career-clinician-educator-year-award.

Chapter 9
Oni Blackstock, MD

Medicine is often described as a small world, and we have all experienced the sparse few degrees of separation between colleagues meeting for the first time at a conference. We do not all know each other—the million strong of the physician workforce is large enough to prevent that—but so often the much smaller key voices of our number connect the collective. They are friends, mentors, leaders, advocates; the hinge points of our networks who compel innovation whenever the gears of medicine begin to show rust. As a student, I also found that these voices so eloquently described the faults of medicine, even as they illuminated its successes, in balanced but forthright ways that rallied the burgeoning spirit of advocacy within me. By having encountered their words and work, I find, now, that I am a better physician. Dr. Oni Blackstock is one such voice, whose research advocacy remains an inspiration.

Dr. Oni Blackstock was born on November 4th, 1977, in Brooklyn, New York, alongside her fraternal twin sister, Uché [1, 2]. From the very beginning, the Blackstock twins were destined for medicine, though not in the prescriptive way that some physician families might impose such a path. Rather, theirs was a legacy born of witnessing their mother's joy and purpose, of accompanying Dr. Dale Gloria Blackstock to community health fairs throughout Brooklyn, of watching her educate neighbors about kidney disease and hypertension with the same warmth she showed her own daughters [3]. Dale Blackstock had evaded poverty through education, becoming the first in her family to attend college, and then defying a nun who told her she could only aspire to be a teacher by earning admission to Harvard Medical School [1, 4]. She returned to the very Brooklyn neighborhood where she'd grown up on welfare, where she'd put cardboard in her shoes when the soles wore through, and she spent her career as a nephrologist serving those communities [2, 3]. She became president of a Black women physicians' group in Brooklyn, and for young Oni and Uché, it seemed that most doctors were Black women, until college revealed the stark reality that Black women physicians comprise less than 3% of all physicians in America [1, 5].

O. M. Cox, *The Pen, The Stethoscope, and The Scalpel*,
https://doi.org/10.1007/978-3-032-19406-0_9

The summer after Oni's sophomore year at Harvard, where she was studying computer science on a full scholarship, Dr. Dale Blackstock died of leukemia at age 47 [1, 3]. Years later, Uché would explore in her book "Legacy: A Black Physician Reckons with Racism in Medicine," how their mother's death might have been connected to growing up near one of four radioactive dumping grounds in New York City, two of which were situated in predominantly Black and Latinx communities [3, 4]. The loss crystallized for the twins what their mother had always known: that health outcomes are inseparable from social context, that the ZIP code in which you're born can determine how long you live, and that being a physician means confronting the systems that create these inequities.

I discovered Dr. Blackstock's work during my own medical training, in that peculiar way that important voices find you when you need them most. I was grappling with questions about how to practice medicine that addressed not just the pathophysiology in front of me but the structural violence that brought my patients through the door. On Twitter, which was then the vibrant ecosystem we called #MedTwitter, I encountered Dr. Blackstock's clear-eyed analysis of the HIV epidemic in New York City. She wrote about women prioritizing everyone else's health over their own, about cisgender and transgender women facing intersecting oppressions that placed them at highest risk for HIV, about how you cannot end an epidemic without addressing racism, sexism, homophobia, and transphobia. Her voice was neither strident nor performative but rather carried the authority of someone who had seen the data, treated the patients, and understood that clinical excellence alone would never be enough.

Dr. Blackstock's path through medicine reveals the thoughtfulness with which she approached her calling. After Harvard Medical School, she trained in primary care internal medicine at Montefiore Medical Center and Albert Einstein College of Medicine, where she served as ambulatory care chief resident [6, 7]. She completed an HIV clinical fellowship at Harlem Hospital Center, then entered the prestigious Robert Wood Johnson Foundation Clinical Scholars Program at Yale School of Medicine, earning her Master of Health Sciences [6–8]. But prior any of that, immediately after medical school, she traveled to Ghana and South Africa to conduct HIV research [3, 7]. What she witnessed abroad—the devastating disparities in treatment for different demographics—she recognized when she returned home. The same patterns of inequity that denied antiretroviral therapy to Africans manifested in American cities, where Black and Latino communities bore disproportionate burdens of HIV infection while facing barriers to prevention and treatment.

For over 14 years, Dr. Blackstock worked as an HIV physician in New York City, primarily at Harlem Hospital Center where she continues to practice as an attending physician today [9, 10]. Her research focused relentlessly on improving engagement in HIV treatment and prevention services, particularly for women and other marginalized groups [6, 11]. She understood that women often serve as family caregivers and consequently defer their own healthcare needs. She saw mothers bringing their children to clinic appointments, elderly relatives in tow, everyone's health addressed except their own. Her NIH- and CDC-funded research developed and tested interventions that met women where they were, that acknowledged the full complexity of their lives rather than expecting them to fit neatly into protocols designed without their input [6, 8].

In 2017, the Centers for Disease Control awarded Dr. Blackstock a Minority HIV/AIDS Research Initiative grant to improve HIV prevention in at-risk communities. Her project partnered with the New York Harm Reduction Educators organization to focus on women in East Harlem and the Bronx [7]. Through this work, she identified a troubling gap: CDC guidelines for pre-exposure prophylaxis, or PrEP—the highly effective HIV prevention medication—inadvertently disqualified many at-risk women from receiving it [11]. The guidelines had been written without sufficient consideration of women's experiences, and Dr. Blackstock's research illuminated how policy could perpetuate the very inequities it ostensibly sought to address. She wrote about this in Mayo Clinic Proceedings, in an article titled "Preexposure Prophylaxis Is for Women, Too," arguing that the medical establishment needed to reimagine PrEP provision for women entirely [12].

Her qualitative research revealed something crucial about how health information travels through communities: for women, the messenger matters as much as the message. Women who ultimately started PrEP described hearing about it from someone they deeply trusted; a partner, a close friend, a healthcare provider who had taken time to know them [12]. This finding shaped Dr. Blackstock's intervention design, which employed peer educators, cisgender and transgender women who could do outreach and counseling within their own communities, linking women to clinics that actually welcomed them. The intervention offered not just PrEP appointments but referrals for mental health services, housing assistance, and other needs, recognizing that HIV risk doesn't exist in isolation from the rest of life's circumstances.

In 2018, Dr. Blackstock was appointed Assistant Commissioner for the Bureau of HIV at the New York City Department of Health and Mental Hygiene [6, 8]. She led all programmatic and administrative activities for the bureau while maintaining her clinical practice and academic appointment at Montefiore Medical Center and Albert Einstein College of Medicine. Under her leadership, the bureau launched the "Living Sure" campaign, encouraging women to develop sexual health plans. She promoted PrEP to communities worst impacted by the HIV epidemic—women of color, LGBTQ+ individuals—stewarding 23 million dollars into eight clinics across New York City to provide low-cost and no-cost testing and treatment [13]. She spearheaded the "Made Equal" campaign as part of the city's Undetectable equals Untransmittable initiative, spreading the scientifically validated message that people with undetectable HIV viral loads cannot sexually transmit the virus [14]. In 2019, thanks to these comprehensive public health interventions that Dr. Blackstock had initiated and promoted, New York City announced a 67% decline in new HIV diagnoses since 2001 [3, 13, 15]. It was a stunning achievement, the kind of population-level impact that physicians dream of making.

But Dr. Blackstock understood that technical interventions, no matter how well-designed, would always be insufficient without addressing the systems that create health inequities in the first place. When Dr. Mary Bassett, then New York State Health Commissioner, founded the "Race to Justice" initiative to address racism's impacts both within the health department and in the communities it served, Dr. Blackstock started the first bureau-based racial equity and social justice program at the NYC Health Department [3, 9]. She led efforts to improve data equity, enhance health information systems, increase workforce diversity, and foster more equitable administrative and programmatic policies [8]. This work required examining the department's own practices, acknowledging how institutional racism could operate even within an agency dedicated to public health, and creating structures for ongoing accountability.

Then came COVID-19, and everything changed. In the early months of 2020, as the pandemic devastated New York City, Dr. Blackstock found herself leading a 300-person bureau through the unprecedented crisis [3]. She made the wrenching decision to pull her entire team from community-facing work, a profound shift for an organization built around meeting people where they were. They had to innovate rapidly, finding ways to reach communities virtually even as those same communities were being decimated by coronavirus. Dr. Blackstock worked 7 days a week, often around the clock, witnessing how the virus exposed and amplified every existing inequity [3]. Black and Latino New Yorkers were dying at dramatically higher rates than white residents. The causes were layered and intersecting: higher rates of underlying health conditions stemming from chronic stress and limited healthcare access, greater likelihood of working essential jobs with public exposure, living in multigenerational housing that made isolation impossible, hospitals in their neighborhoods that were under-resourced and overwhelmed, and provider bias that meant their symptoms were taken less seriously.

In April 2020, Mother Jones magazine featured the Blackstock twins as being "on the front lines of New York City's fight against the coronavirus pandemic [13]." Dr. Oni Blackstock called COVID-19 a "pandemic of inequality," a phrase that captured what we were all witnessing but struggled to articulate [13, 16]. She and her team at the NYC Health Department created guidance on practicing safe sex during the pandemic; advice that went viral for its frank acknowledgment that people would continue to have intimate lives even during lockdown [3]. "You are your safest sex partner," the guidance began, before moving to partners you live with, then discussing how to reduce risk with others [13]. It was classic Dr. Blackstock: pragmatic, nonjudgmental, meeting people where they were rather than where public health officials wished they would be. She also provided specific guidance for New Yorkers living with HIV, addressing how the pandemic intersected with their existing health concerns and how to protect themselves while maintaining their HIV care.

The pandemic crystallized something for Dr. Blackstock that had been building throughout her career. Despite working within the NYC Health Department, she realized that the most transformative work might happen outside such structures, where she could have more control over her time, her approach, and her collaborations. In August 2020, even as she continued to lead the city's COVID response, she founded Health Justice, a consulting firm dedicated to helping health-related organizations center antiracism and equity in their workplaces while reducing health inequities in the communities they serve [3, 8].

Health Justice represents the culmination of Dr. Blackstock's career trajectory, drawing on her clinical expertise, her research methodology, her public health leadership, and yes, even her undergraduate computer science training [8]. The firm works with healthcare systems, public health departments, and nonprofits to assess racial equity through data gathered via interviews, focus groups, and surveys about organizational culture, commitment, and programming [3]. They run sessions with executive teams to ensure leadership ownership of equity goals, because transformation cannot succeed if it's delegated to a diversity officer while executives continue unchanged. Dr. Blackstock designs microlearning courses that organizations can complete independently, and she gives talks about her career trajectory and her approach to community-centered, participatory, inclusive healthcare. Upcoming courses address artificial intelligence and large language models; those computer science courses from her Harvard days proved unexpectedly relevant to ensuring that emerging technologies don't replicate or amplify existing biases [3].

In just 4 years, Health Justice has worked with over 100 clients across the country, including Salesforce, Northwestern Lurie Children's Hospital—where I completed my residency—and Partners HealthCare System [8]. Dr. Blackstock attributes much of her success to her reputation and professional network, the relationships she'd formed through decades of clinical practice, research, and public health work. But there's something else at play too: her lived experience at the intersection of multiple marginalized identities—Black, woman, lesbian, daughter of a mother who died too young from a disease potentially linked to environmental racism—gives her both insight and authority [8, 9]. She doesn't speak about health equity from theory alone; she speaks from having navigated systems that were not designed for her, from having cared for patients facing similar navigation, from having transformed those systems from the inside and now working to change them from the outside.

Dr. Blackstock maintains her clinical practice at Harlem Hospital Center, seeing patients, staying grounded in the daily reality of providing care [9]. This commitment to remaining a practicing physician even while running Health Justice speaks to her understanding that credibility in health equity work requires ongoing clinical engagement. You cannot advocate for patients if you've lost touch with the realities of their daily lives, with which barriers they continually face, and with how policy translates to the exam room. Her approach embodies what she calls "structural humility [8, 9];" recognizing that health inequities are rooted in systemic factors, being open to learning from those directly impacted, and reflecting constantly on whether one's actions perpetuate or help alleviate inequity.

The Blackstock sisters have become prominent voices in healthcare, their twinship adding a unique dimension to their impact. They appear together frequently—at conferences, on podcasts, in interviews—where their distinct yet complementary perspectives illuminate different facets of health equity work. Uché, an emergency medicine physician and founder of Advancing Health Equity, focuses her consulting practice similarly on dismantling structural racism in healthcare [1]. When they speak together, you sense the foundation of shared experience: the mother who inspired them, the Harvard education they both received, the choice they both made to return to New York City to serve communities like the one in which they were raised. Yet you also see their individual contributions: Oni's HIV and primary care focus, her public health systems expertise, her research methodology; Uché's emergency medicine acumen, her academic leadership, her willingness to name racism explicitly even when it costs her professionally.

In 2019, Out magazine honored Dr. Blackstock for her efforts to end the HIV epidemic, recognizing her work promoting PrEP to LGBTQ+ communities and championing the U=U message that gave HIV-positive individuals scientific backing for their lived knowledge that they couldn't transmit the virus when their viral load was undetectable [14]. Essence magazine featured her as a Black mom on the front lines of healthcare [2]. Marie Claire and other publications profiled her health equity work. She has appeared on CNN, MSNBC, Good Morning America, and Democracy Now!, translating complex public health concepts into accessible language while never shying from uncomfortable truths about racism in medicine [8].

On Twitter, where I first encountered her work, Dr. Blackstock built a significant following by sharing her insights on health equity, responding to followers' questions, and providing real-time analysis of developing public health issues. During the pandemic, her Twitter threads offered crucial information to communities receiving mixed messages from official sources. She exemplified how physicians can use social media not for self-promotion but for genuine public health communication, meeting people in the digital spaces they already inhabit. Her willingness to be accessible, to engage with critiques and questions, to acknowledge uncertainty while providing the best available evidence, modeled the kind of physician-communicator our increasingly complex health landscape requires.

Dr. Blackstock has published extensively in peer-reviewed journals on topics ranging from PrEP awareness among Black and Latina women to the role of structural racism in HIV outcomes to health justice as a framework for addressing COVID-19's disproportionate impacts [8]. Her article "Health Justice: A Framework for Mitigating the Impacts of HIV and COVID-19 on Disproportionately Affected Communities" articulated how interconnected oppressions create and sustain health inequities, and how interventions must be equally comprehensive to succeed [17]. She has written about past as prologue; how colonial legacies must be dismantled to advance Black health equity in the United States. She has called healthcare "the new battlefront for anti-DEI attacks," warning that efforts to eliminate diversity, equity, and inclusion initiatives will harm patients, particularly those from marginalized communities who already face barriers to quality care [18].

Though Dr. Blackstock has not authored a book of her own—her sister Uché published "Legacy: A Black Physician Reckons with Racism in Medicine" in 2024, a powerful memoir that tells their mother's story and examines systemic racism in healthcare [1, 4]—her impact on medical literature comes through her research articles, op-eds, keynote addresses, and the tangible policy changes her work has generated. She has influenced how we think about PrEP for women, how we structure HIV prevention programs, how health departments can operate with equity as a core principle, and how organizations across healthcare can begin the long work of antiracism. These contributions may not sit on bookstore shelves, but they shape practice guidelines, inform training curricula, and ultimately save lives.

In interviews, Dr. Blackstock speaks about learning to extend herself grace, to see setbacks as learning opportunities rather than failures. She describes how perfectionistic she can be, how hard she is on herself, and how she's had to cultivate a mindset of perpetual learning rather than achieved mastery [8]. This humility feels essential to equity work, which by definition requires ongoing self-examination and willingness to be wrong. If you think you've "solved" racism or achieved perfect antiracism, you've misunderstood the assignment. The work is generational, iterative, uncomfortable, and never finished. Dr. Blackstock models how to sustain yourself in such work without either burnout or complacency; by staying connected to clinical practice, by building community with others doing similar work, by celebrating incremental victories while remaining clear-eyed about the distance still to travel. She also speaks about the importance of building relationships before you need them, of how Health Justice's rapid growth stemmed partly from professional networks she'd cultivated throughout her career [8].

Dr. Blackstock's story also illuminates the particular challenges and opportunities of being a physician of color, especially a Black woman physician. She navigates predominantly white spaces where her expertise is questioned in ways white colleagues' expertise never is. She faces the emotional labor of explaining structural racism to audiences who'd rather believe the playing field is level. She carries the weight of patients who seek her out specifically because they've been harmed by provider bias and hope a Black physician will actually listen to them. She manages the impossibility of being expected to fix centuries of systemic oppression while receiving a fraction of the resources and support that white-led initiatives receive. Yet she also brings perspective that comes from lived experience, understands barriers intimately because she or her loved ones have faced them, and can build trust with communities that have every reason to distrust medical institutions.

She is a mother, she has said, and like many working mothers, she tries to protect her children from negative messages about their worth. She tapes daily affirmations to her bathroom mirror, telling her sons they are valued, they are worthy, they are loved. This is the other pandemic she faces, the one that predated COVID-19 and will outlast it: the pandemic of racist messages that tell Black children, especially Black boys, that they are threatening, expendable, less-than [10]. She works to transform healthcare systems while simultaneously protecting her own children's spirits, to dismantle structural barriers while building her sons' sense of self. The personal is never separate from the professional when you live at the intersection of marginalized identities.

As I write this essay, I think about what Dr. Blackstock's voice has meant to me personally. She provided evidence for what I felt intuitively; that you cannot separate illness from the conditions that produce it, that medical expertise without structural competency is incomplete, that the most impactful interventions often happen outside the clinic. She modeled how to be rigorous and compassionate simultaneously, how to critique systems while caring for individuals within them, how to maintain hope without naivety.

Dr. Oni Blackstock's legacy is still being written. The organizations she has consulted with, the policies she has shaped, the research that will cite her work, the physicians she has influenced (including, humbly, myself); these ripple effects extend far beyond what can be measured. But if there is a through-line to her career, it is this: that health equity requires clinical excellence combined with structural competency, individual compassion alongside policy change, research rigor plus community partnership. It requires physicians who remember why they went into medicine in the first place; not to uphold existing systems but to serve patients, all patients, especially those whom systems have failed.

References

1. Harvard Medicine Magazine. Family. n.d. https://magazine.hms.harvard.edu/articles/family.
2. Essence. Black moms on the front lines: Twin doctors Uché and Oni Blackstock are battling structural racism in medicine for Black lives. 2020, May 22. https://www.essence.com/feature/black-moms-front-lines-twin-doctors-uche-oni-blackstock-battling-structural-racism-in-medicine/.
3. Harvard John A. Paulson School of Engineering and Applied Sciences. Alumni profile: Oni Blackstock, A.B. '99, MD '05. 2024, December 11. https://seas.harvard.edu/news/2024/12/alumni-profile-oni-blackstock-ab-99-md-05.
4. Harvard Gazette. Excerpt from 'Legacy' by Uché Blackstock. 2024, February. https://news.harvard.edu/gazette/story/2024/02/was-racism-a-risk-factor-in-mothers-leukemia/.
5. Marketplace. A physician explores the obstacles keeping Black people out of medicine. 2024, January 25. https://www.marketplace.org/story/2024/01/25/physician-explores-obstacles-keeping-black-americans-out-of-medicine.
6. Yale Center for Interdisciplinary Research on AIDS (CIRA). Oni Blackstock, M.D. n.d. https://cira.yale.edu/people/oni-blackstock-md.
7. National Coalition of STD Directors (NCSD). Black History Month blog: Dr. Oni Blackstock, health equity champion. 2020, March 6. https://ncsddc.org/black-history-month-blog-dr-oni-blackstock-health-equity-champion/.
8. Health Justice. About. n.d. https://www.healthjustice.co/about/
9. NPR Diverse Sources Database. Oni Blackstock. 2022, July 17. https://training.npr.org/sources/oni-blackstock/.
10. Fougere D, Cabana J. Twin sisters, both doctors, take on health care inequality. NY1. 2023, February 28. https://ny1.com/nyc/all-boroughs/news/2023/02/28/twin-sisters%2D%2Dboth-doctors%2D%2Dbattle-health-care-inequalities.
11. AIDSVu. Dr. Oni Blackstock on HIV among women and vulnerable populations. 2019, March 7. https://aidsvu.org/news-updates/oni-blackstock-hiv-women-vulnerable/.
12. Blackstock OJ. Preexposure prophylaxis is for women, too. Mayo Clin Proc. 2018;93(3):395–6. https://doi.org/10.1016/j.mayocp.2017.12.005.
13. Regis College. The equalizer: Q&A with Dr. Oni Blackstock. n.d. https://www.regiscollege.edu/about-regis/news/equalizer-qa-dr-oni-blackstock.
14. Out. These Out100 honorees are doing the work to end the HIV epidemic. 2019, November 23. https://www.out.com/print/2019/11/23/out100-ending-hiv-gareth-thomas-steven-thrasher-demetre-blackstock.
15. News-Medical. HIV diagnosis falls to a record low in NYC, finds report. 2019, November 25. https://www.news-medical.net/news/20191125/HIV-diagnosis-falls-to-a-record-low-in-NYC-finds-report.aspx.

16. STAT News. STATUS List: Oni Blackstock. 2022, February 19. https://www.statnews.com/status-list/2022/oni-blackstock/.
17. Alang S, Blackstock O. Health justice: a framework for mitigating the impacts of HIV and COVID-19 on disproportionately affected communities. Am J Public Health. 2023;113(2):194–201. https://doi.org/10.2105/AJPH.2022.307139.
18. Blackstock OJ, Isom JE, Legha RK. Health care is the new battlefront for anti-DEI attacks. PLOS Global Public Health. 2024;4(4):e0003131. https://doi.org/10.1371/journal.pgph.0003131.

Chapter 10
Jennifer Gunter, MD

In my second year of medical school, one of our lecturers, an OB-GYN, led a week-long session on health concerns primarily related to or affecting individuals with uteruses. This, it would turn out, would be our only dedicated pre-clinical opportunity to review pathophysiology and clinical logistics affecting, primarily women. It was also noted to be an improvement upon what had been a single day of learning, in response to advocacy by student leaders in the school's chapter of Medical Students for Choice. In retrospect, our school was not alone in accepting this brief review as sufficient for medical students. A 2008 study by Henrich et al. on medical student perceptions of women's health teaching, found that most students assessed their curricula on women's health as moderate at best, while simultaneously expressing confidence in their ability to manage women's health issues [1]. In 2016, Jenkins et al. published a similar study and found that fewer than half (48.1%) the medical students surveyed agreed that they had specific classes or programs on sex and gender differences, and less than a third (31.1%) reported that a sex and gender-based curriculum existed within their medical school. Numerous studies have expounded upon the reasons for a dearth of knowledge on women's health, often highlighting historical exclusion from clinical trials [2]. Also in 2016, the National Institutes of Health stated that future grants funded by the collaborative, would be required to have sex included as a biological variable in study design [3]. This milestone, notwithstanding, the gulf of knowledge on women's health remains vast. It is why I am appreciative of physicians such as Dr. Jennifer Gunter, whose pen and prose work faster than governmental policies are implemented.

Dr. Jennifer Gunter was born on September 7th, 1966, in Winnipeg, Manitoba, Canada, into what would become a story of medical calling rooted in childhood trauma and curiosity [4, 5]. When she was 11 years old, a skateboard accident sent her to the hospital with a ruptured spleen [6]. In that moment—injured, scared, a child facing her own fragility—Dr. Gunter made a choice that would define her career. She declined sedation. Instead, she watched, transfixed, as the medical team performed an angiogram on her ruptured spleen, explaining each step of the

O. M. Cox, *The Pen, The Stethoscope, and The Scalpel*,
https://doi.org/10.1007/978-3-032-19406-0_10

procedure as they worked. Most children would have turned away, sought comfort in unconsciousness, but Dr. Gunter leaned in.[11] She wanted to understand what was happening to her body, wanted to witness the mechanics of healing, wanted to know. That curiosity—the refusal to look away from difficult truths combined with an insistence on understanding rather than accepting—became the foundation of everything that followed.

From 1984 to 1986, Dr. Gunter studied at the University of Winnipeg before being accepted into medical school at age 20 [5]. In 1990, at just 23 years old, she graduated from the University of Manitoba College of Medicine [4, 5]. I pause here to note that she was 23 when she earned her medical degree, an age when many of us are still figuring out what we wanted to be. From 1990 to 1995, she completed obstetrics and gynecology training at the University of Western Ontario in London, Ontario [4, 5]. In 1995, Dr. Gunter moved to the United States for a fellowship in infectious diseases and women's health at the University of Kansas Medical Center, where she also developed an interest in pain management [4, 5].

The trajectory seemed straightforward: a young Canadian physician building an academic career in the United States, specializing in OB-GYN, perhaps destined for a quiet life of clinical practice and teaching. But life, as it does, intervened with devastating force. In 2001, while working as a lecturer at the University of Colorado Hospital in Denver, Dr. Gunter became pregnant with triplets [6, 7]. At 22 weeks and 3 days, her water broke. She went to the hospital convinced she would lose all three boys. What happened instead was a trauma that would reshape her entire career. After nearly 2 days of labor, she delivered her first son, Aidan [7]. He weighed one pound. He died shortly after birth. The image of watching her son die—a physician unable to save her own child, a mother witnessing the unbearable—caused Dr. Gunter to give up obstetrics entirely [7]. She could no longer deliver babies, could no longer be in that space where joy and devastation exist in such close proximity. Her two other sons, Victor and Oliver, were delivered at 26 weeks and survived, but faced severe health complications. Both boys had lung disease secondary to prematurity and required oxygen for a year, particularly in the setting of Denver's high altitude and consequent decreased partial pressure of oxygen [7].

It was during this nightmare period, sitting up late at night with her premature infants, that Dr. Gunter first encountered the vast ocean of medical misinformation available to desperate parents. She was a physician—board-certified, highly trained, evidence-based in her approach—and even she struggled to separate facts from fiction in the overwhelming amount of information about premature babies available online [7]. The experience was radicalizing. If she, with all her medical training, found it difficult to navigate the misinformation, how did everyone else manage? What were her own patients encountering when they Googled their symptoms at two in the morning? She started to see the bad information her patients brought to the office in a new light. It wasn't ignorance or gullibility; it was the predictable result of a medical internet polluted with pseudoscience, celebrity endorsements, and fearmongering designed to sell products.

The loss of Aidan transformed Dr. Gunter's practice in another way. She shifted her focus from obstetrics to gynecology, specializing in vaginal and vulval conditions, particularly chronic pelvic pain and vulvodynia [7]. These are conditions often dismissed by other physicians, conditions where women are told the pain is in their heads, where suffering is minimized or pathologized. Dr. Gunter became board-certified in pain medicine by both the American Board of Pain Medicine and the American Board of Physical Medicine and Rehabilitation. (Hence the impressive string of letters after her name: MD, FRCS(C), FACOG, DABPM, ABPMR.) [4] Although her career in the States had started in Kansas, and continued in Colorado, in 2006, she moved to California, and has been at The Permanente Medical Group of Kaiser Permanente in Northern California, ever since [7, 8]. This decision was partly driven by the closer proximity to sea level that the West Coast offered, compared to Denver [7].

Her first book, "The Preemie Primer: A Complete Guide for Parents of Premature Babies – from Birth through the Toddler Years and Beyond," was published in 2010 [6]. It was born directly from her experience with Victor and Oliver, a guide she wished had existed when she needed it most [7]. The book provided medically sound, accessible information for parents navigating the terrifying world of neonatal intensive care. But it was what came next that would make Dr. Gunter a household name, at least in households that follow healthcare Twitter drama.

In 2011, Dr. Gunter started a blog. By 2017, it had reached 15 million views and generated considerable controversy in mainstream media [9, 10]. She wrote about reproductive health, vaccination, evidence-based medicine, and the careless way media outlets reported on these topics [4]. She took on dubious health claims made by celebrities. She was critical, acerbic, and unafraid. Her blog became a destination for people seeking reliable information about women's health, and a thorn in the side of anyone peddling pseudoscience.

Then came the jade eggs. In January 2017, Gwyneth Paltrow's lifestyle brand Goop published an interview with "beauty guru/healer/inspiration/friend" Shiva Rose about jade and rose quartz eggs that women could insert into their vaginas [11]. According to Goop, these eggs—priced at 55–66 dollars—would help "cultivate sexual energy, increase orgasm, balance the cycle, stimulate key reflexology around vaginal walls, tighten and tone, prevent uterine prolapse, increase control of the whole perineum and bladder, develop and clear chi pathways in the body, intensify feminine energy," and were marketed as an ancient practice of "Chinese concubines and royalty [7]." The claims were extraordinary. The evidence was nonexistent.

On January 17, 2017, Dr. Gunter published a blog post titled "Dear Gwyneth Paltrow, I'm a GYN and your vaginal jade eggs are a bad idea [4]." The post went viral. "I've been reading all about the jade eggs you are selling on Goop for $55-66 a pop," Dr. Gunter wrote. She methodically dismantled every claim. Jade is porous, she explained, which could allow bacteria to colonize the stone, potentially leading to bacterial vaginosis or toxic shock syndrome. The idea that these eggs were used by Chinese royalty was historically dubious. Dr. Gunter later co-authored a peer-reviewed paper with Egyptologist Sarah Parcak titled "Vaginal Jade Eggs: Ancient

Chinese Practice or Modern Marketing Myth?" in which they confirmed that no archaeological or historical evidence supported this claim [12]. As for the muscular benefits, Dr. Gunter pointed out that overenthusiastic or incorrectly performed Kegel exercises are a cause of pelvic pain and painful sex in her practice. "Imagine how your biceps muscle (and then your shoulders and then your back) might feel if you walked around all day flexed holding a barbell? Right, now imagine your pelvic floor muscles doing this [13]."

The post was picked up by tabloid newspapers, then by major media outlets. CNN, Gizmodo, The Washington Post, all quoted Dr. Gunter's critique. It was a bad news day for Goop, and presumably not great for sales. In July 2017, Goop struck back, publishing a piece by contributors Steven Gundry and Aviva Romm that attacked Dr. Gunter personally, questioning her expertise and accusing her of bullying women who found alternative practices helpful. The piece was titled "A Note From Dr. Steven Gundry" and began by questioning Dr. Gunter's parenting skills, saying "…a very wise Professor of Surgery at the University of Michigan once instructed me to never write anything that my mother or child wouldn't be proud to read [14]." Gwyneth Paltrow herself tweeted the article, quoting Michelle Obama: "When they go low, we go high [14]."

The medical and scientific community rallied to Dr. Gunter's defense. Dr. Jennifer Raff tweeted, "Dear @goop, We stand behind @DrJenGunter and we support her in calling out your nonsense. Sincerely, Science twitter [15]." The controversy catapulted Dr. Gunter to wider fame. Her blog traffic tripled between 2013 and 2016, and the Goop response drove her 2017 traffic to an all-time high of six million views. Editors from BuzzFeed, The Atlantic, and The New York Times took notice.

In September 2018, Goop agreed to pay $145,000 in civil penalties to settle a consumer protection lawsuit brought by the Santa Clara County District Attorney's Office and nine other California prosecutors [16]. The suit specifically cited "unsupported attributes for Goop's Jade Egg, Rose Quartz Egg, and Inner Judge Flower Essence Blend." The company agreed to refund customers who purchased the products and to stop advertising them as remedies for health ailments [15]. Dr. Gunter had won, at least in the court of law. In the court of public opinion, the battle continued.

Dr. Gunter didn't want to build a career out of criticizing Goop, but Goop kept providing material. When the brand launched a Netflix series called "The Goop Lab" in January 2020, featuring episodes on exorcisms, psychedelics, psychic mediums, and energy healing, Dr. Gunter told people to read her book "The Vagina Bible before watching," so they could separate fact from fiction. "I'd just write it off as crazy except some people are going to follow this advice and waste a lot of money," she wrote [17].

"The Vagina Bible" Published in 2019, the book became an instant #1 Canadian bestseller and a New York Times bestseller [4, 18]. The full title "The Vagina Bible: The Vulva and the Vagina – Separating the Myth from the Medicine," captures Dr. Gunter's mission perfectly. The book is comprehensive, covering reproductive health, the impact of antibiotics and probiotics, vaginal steaming, marijuana products for vaginal use, period products, sexually transmitted infections, contraception, menstruation, and menopause. It includes a section on transgender men and women, acknowledging that not everyone with a vagina identifies as a woman. The tone is conversational yet authoritative, evidence-based yet empathetic. It's the book Dr. Gunter wished existed when she was in medical training, the book her patients needed when they came to her with questions their previous doctors had dismissed [4, 18].

The book's promotion generated its own controversy. Twitter initially blocked advertisements for the book because they contained the word "vagina," which the platform deemed inappropriate. The incident highlighted the very problem Dr. Gunter was fighting: the stigma around female anatomy was so pervasive that even the anatomically correct name for a body part was considered obscene. After public outcry, Twitter reversed its decision [19].

In 2021, Dr. Gunter published "The Menopause Manifesto: Own Your Health with Facts and Feminism [4, 20]." The subtitle alone is a mission statement. Like "The Vagina Bible," it became a New York Times bestseller, USA Today bestseller, Washington Post bestseller, and San Francisco Chronicle bestseller [4]. The book counters myths about menopause with evidence-based medicine, historical perspective, and expert advice. Dr. Gunter tackles hot flashes, sleep disruption, sex and libido, depression, skin and hair changes, breast health, outdated therapies, and health maintenance. She is particularly critical of bioidentical hormones, which are often marketed by celebrities as "natural" alternatives to hormone replacement therapy but lack the regulation and testing of FDA-approved treatments [20].

The book was lauded by fellow physicians and by women desperate for reliable information. "Gunter, a specialist in obstetrics and gynecology, follows up the best-selling The Vagina Bible with another essential book on women's health," wrote Library Journal in a starred review, adding [21], "Like her previous guide, Gunter's latest book will find a wide audience, with its clear writing and up-to-date research." Publishers Weekly praised her willingness to call out "ineffective and possibly dangerous menopause remedies she sees celebrities hawking," noting that she provides "a great service to readers having trouble sorting through their choices [20, 21]." Dr. Jennifer Lincoln wrote, "This is the new 'it' book for women who want to prepare for or understand what menopause is (and isn't) [20]." The North American Menopause Society gave Dr. Gunter their 2020 NAMS Media Award for her work [20].

In 2024, Dr. Gunter published "Blood: The Science, Medicine, and Mythology of Menstruation [22, 23]." The book examines the menstrual cycle through the lens of science and social justice, exploring how the patriarchy has weaponized menstruation to control and shame women. She discusses period products, menstrual health, the medicalization of normal cycles, and the way menstruation has been stigmatized across cultures. It's yet another area where evidence-based information is desperately needed and often unavailable.

Beyond her books, Dr. Gunter writes a monthly column for The New York Times called "The Cycle" and a weekly column called "You Asked." Her writing has appeared in Glamour, The Cut, USA Today, The Hill, Self, and The New Republic.

She hosts "Jensplaining," a CBC/Amazon Prime docuseries that highlights the impact of medical misinformation on women [4]. She hosts "Body Stuff with Dr. Jen Gunter," a podcast on the TED Audio Collective that launched after her 2020 TED Talk, "Why Can't We Talk About Periods?" received more than two million views in its first 6 months. She also writes The Vajenda, a Substack newsletter that serves as an evidence-based hub for reproductive health [4].

On Twitter, where she had earned the nickname "Twitter's Resident Gynecologist" or "the Internet's OB/GYN," Dr. Gunter has amassed over 300,000 followers [23]. She uses the platform to share information about pain management, debunk myths about women's health, call out misinformation, and engage directly with patients' questions. Her tone is sharp, sometimes snarky, always evidence-based. She's been called "strangely confident" by Goop (to which she responded that she was "an appropriately confident expert"), and "the world's most famous – and outspoken – gynecologist," by The Guardian [24].

Not everyone appreciates Dr. Gunter's approach. In 2019, some fellow physicians and feminists criticized her for what they perceived as a lack of humility and for "bullying" women who found alternative practices helpful. An op-ed in Scientific American (later deleted) by science journalist Jennifer Block was titled "Doctors Are Not Gods" and critiqued Dr. Gunter's work by suggesting she dismissed women's lived experiences [25]. The critiques centered on a fundamental tension: Does advocating for evidence-based medicine inherently dismiss women's experiences and agency? Can a physician be both empowering and rigorously scientific?

Dr. Gunter's response was measured. She pointed out that many quotes in the Scientific American piece were cherry-picked and taken out of context. She noted that she refers to herself as an "expert" strategically, particularly when dealing with trolls or adversaries like Goop. "I also used it when I responded to GOOP for calling me strangely confident," she said. "I told them I was an appropriately confident expert." She acknowledged that alternative practices might provide comfort to some women but maintained that comfort doesn't equal efficacy, and that selling unproven products with false health claims is exploitative [24].

The controversy illustrates a larger debate in modern feminism about the role of medical authority versus individual experience, about empowerment through knowledge versus autonomy to choose unproven treatments. Dr. Gunter has always been clear about where she stands: empowerment requires accurate information. You cannot make informed choices if the information you're receiving is false. The wellness industry profits from women's distrust of the medical establishment, a distrust that is often justified given medicine's history of dismissing women's pain and pathologizing female bodies. But the solution isn't to abandon evidence-based medicine for jade eggs and vaginal steaming; it's to reform medicine so that it serves women better, so that evidence-based care is also compassionate care.

Dr. Gunter has devoted her professional life to caring for women, as she often says. She has published extensively in peer-reviewed journals on topics including vulvodynia, chronic pelvic pain, intimate partner violence, and HPV vaccination [4]. She successfully pushed for a retraction and apology from the Toronto Star in 2015 after the newspaper published an article mischaracterizing the safety of the

HPV vaccine Gardasil, leading to broader scrutiny of how mainstream media covers vaccine safety [4, 26]. And her advocacy isn't limited to battling wellness brands or educating patients. It extends to fixing the medical internet more broadly, to creating a body of work that will outlast any single product or celebrity [4].

In the current landscape of medicine, where misinformation spreads faster than fact, where social media algorithms amplify outrage over accuracy, where celebrity endorsements carry more weight than peer-reviewed research, we need more physician-advocates like Dr. Gunter. We need people willing to say unpopular things, to challenge powerful brands, to risk criticism and controversy in service of truth. We need physicians who write for the public, who meet people where they are—on social media, in podcasts, through accessible books—who translate complex medical information into language that empowers rather than intimidates.

But more than that, we need a medical system that doesn't require individual heroes to counter systemic failures. We need medical education that adequately covers women's health, that teaches about vulvovaginal disorders and chronic pelvic pain with the same depth it teaches about cardiac physiology. We need research that includes women, that investigates conditions predominantly affecting women, that doesn't dismiss female pain as psychosomatic. We need healthcare that is accessible, that listens to women's concerns, that treats female patients with the same seriousness as male patients. We need regulation of the wellness industry, enforcement against false health claims, accountability for companies that exploit women's legitimate frustrations with inadequate healthcare.

Until that systemic change happens, we have Dr. Gunter and physicians like her, fighting the good fight, one blog post, one book, one Twitter thread at a time. The work is exhausting, I'm sure. The criticism is relentless. The need is infinite. But someone has to do it.

References

1. Henrich JB, Viscoli CM, Abraham GD. Medical students' assessment of education and training in women's health and in sex and gender differences. J Women's Health. 2008;17(5):815–27. https://doi.org/10.1089/jwh.2007.0589.
2. Jenkins MR, Herrmann A, Tashjian A, Ramineni T, Ramakrishnan R, Raef D, Rokas T, Shatzer J. Sex and gender in medical education: a national student survey. Biol Sex Differ. 2016;7(Suppl 1):45. https://doi.org/10.1186/s13293-016-0094-6.
3. National Institutes of Health. Consideration of sex as a biological variable in NIH-funded research. 2015. https://grants.nih.gov/grants/guide/notice-files/NOT-OD-15-102.html.
4. Gunter J. About me. Dr. Jen Gunter. n.d. https://drjengunter.com/about-me/.
5. Hachette UK. Dr. Jennifer Gunter. n.d. https://www.hachette.co.uk/contributor/dr-jennifer-gunter/.
6. Gunter J. The preemie primer: a complete guide for parents of premature babies. Cambridge: Da Capo Lifelong Books; 2010.
7. Halushak M. Meet Goop's number-one enemy. Chatelaine. 2019, July 16. https://chatelaine.com/health/jen-gunter-profile/.

8. Kaiser Permanente. My doctor online: Jennifer Gunter, MD. n.d. https://mydoctor.kaiserpermanente.org/ncal/doctor/jennifergunter/about.
9. CBC Media Centre. New CBC original docseries, "Jensplaining," hosted by "Twitter's resident gynecologist" Dr. Jen Gunter launches August 23 on CBC Gem. 2019, June 12. https://mediacentre.cbc.ca/announcement/4163/new-cbc-original-docseries-jensplaining-hosted-by-twitter-s-resident-gynecologist-dr-jen-gunter-launches-august-23-on-cbc-gem/.
10. Girvan CE. Debunking the scientifically inaccurate: Dr. Jen Gunter is on a mission for women's health. iPolitics. 2018, July 13. https://web.archive.org/web/20210527032112/ipolitics.ca/article/debunking-the-scientifically-inaccurate-dr-jen-gunter-is-on-a-mission-for-womens-health/.
11. Ross M. SF gynecologist blasts Gwyneth Paltrow for jade eggs for your "yoni" and "toxic" tampon advice. The Mercury News. 2017, January 20. https://www.mercurynews.com/2017/01/20/sf-gynecologist-blasts-gwyneth-paltrow-for-jade-eggs-for-your-yoni-and-tampon-advice/.
12. Gunter J, Parcak S. Vaginal jade eggs: ancient Chinese practice or modern marketing myth? Female Pelvic Med Reconstr Surg. 2019;25(1):1–2. https://doi.org/10.1097/SPV.0000000000000643.
13. Belluz J. Let's call Gwyneth Paltrow's jade eggs for vaginas what they are: Goopshit. Vox. 2017, January 23. https://www.vox.com/policy-and-politics/2017/1/23/14352904/gwyneth-paltrow-jade-eggs.
14. Truong K. What Gwyneth Paltrow has to say to Goop detractors. Refinery29. 2017, July 13. https://www.refinery29.com/en-us/2017/07/163302/gwyneth-paltrow-goop-doctors-response.
15. Sacks B. Gwyneth Paltrow's Goop will pay $145,000 for misleading customers about that vagina egg. BuzzFeed News. 2018, September 5. https://www.buzzfeednews.com/article/briannasacks/goop-vagina-eggs-settlement.
16. Santa Clara County District Attorney's Office. Goop to pay $145,000 in civil penalties. 2018, September 4. https://da.sonomacounty.ca.gov/jill-ravitch-announces-consumer-protection-settlement.
17. Rosman K. A doctor gives Gwyneth Paltrow's Goop an examination. The New York Times. 2017, July 29. https://www.nytimes.com/2017/07/29/style/goop-gwyneth-paltrow-dr-jen--gunter.html.
18. Gunter J. The vagina bible: the vulva and the vagina—separating the myth from the medicine. New York: Citadel Press; 2019.
19. Rannard G. The Vagina Bible adverts blocked by social media. BBC. 2019, August 30. https://www.bbc.com/news/blogs-trending-49500822.
20. Gunter J. The menopause manifesto: own your health with facts and feminism. New York: Citadel Press/Kensington Publishing Corp; 2021.
21. Library Journal. The Menopause Manifesto: own your health with facts and feminism [Review]. 2021. https://www.libraryjournal.com/review/the-menopause-manifesto-own-your-health-with-facts-and-feminism.
22. Gunter J. Blood. New York, NY. Citadel Press; 2024.
23. Gunter J. [@DrJenGunter]. Tweets [X profile]. X. n.d.. https://x.com/DrJenGunter.
24. Wiseman E. Jennifer Gunter: "Women are being told lies about their bodies." The Guardian 2019, September 8. https://www.theguardian.com/lifeandstyle/2019/sep/08/jennifer-gunter-gynaecologist-womens-health-bodies-myths-and-medicine.
25. Block J. Doctors are not gods. Sci Am. 2019, November 26. https://www.scientificamerican.com/blog/observations/doctors-are-not-gods/.
26. English K. Public editor criticizes the Star's Gardasil story. Toronto Star. 2015, February 14. https://www.thestar.com/opinion/public-editor/public-editor-criticizes-the-stars-gardasil-story/article_56f752dd-b14b-5c4f-b243-f342b94766ee.html.

Chapter 11
Christine Montross, MD

The rite of passage that is the anatomy lab in medical school is necessarily borne with some trepidation and an almost unwilling fascination. For many, it was our first encounter with a person in a state of death. Illness we had likely confronted; whether it was within ourselves or in our loved ones. It also marked the beginning of what would be a system-based exploration of anatomy and pathophysiology. And at the end, a ceremony to honor our still, quiet teachers, attended, often, by their living relatives. In retrospect, I am most struck by our lack of conversation about the time we spent in the lab. Unlike other classes, and with the exception of specific academic inquiries, we rarely discussed the time we spent in the chilled, fluorescent hall. Perhaps it was an act of respect, but I wonder if we could have put in words the emotions between our first and last incisions. "Body of Work" is that cathartic exercise, which we may all need; Dr. Christine Montross illustrates the many sentiments we have, some of us, locked away. It is my honor to share her work with you.

Dr. Christine Elaine Montross was born in 1973 in Indianapolis, Indiana, to Scott and Janice Montross [1]. She grew up in a household where both athleticism and intellectual pursuit were valued; her brother, Eric Montross, would go on to play in the NBA and become a sports commentator [2, 3], while Christine herself gravitated toward literature and the natural world [1, 3]. From early on, hers was a path defined not by straight lines but by winding roads, by the accumulation of seemingly disparate interests that would eventually converge in her work as a physician-writer.

In retrospect, it seems almost inevitable that Montross would become both doctor and author, but the journey there was anything but linear. She attended the She attended the University of Michigan, where she studied French literature and environmental science as an undergraduate [1, 4, 5]. Although these two were seemingly disparate, both required close observation, careful attention to detail, an appreciation for the beautiful and the complex. Both demanded that she look at the world with open eyes and ask: what is this? Why does it matter? How does it work?

O. M. Cox, *The Pen, The Stethoscope, and The Scalpel*,
https://doi.org/10.1007/978-3-032-19406-0_11

After graduating in 1996, Montross remained at the University of Michigan to pursue a Master of Fine Arts in poetry, which she completed in 1998 [5]. During her graduate studies, her poems were published in literary journals including Calyx, Witness, and Alligator Juniper [6, 7]. She taught writing classes as a lecturer at the university [7]. She met her wife, Deborah Salem Smith, a playwright, and the two moved to San Francisco together [2, 8]. It was there, teaching high school English at a charter school for at-risk students, that something shifted. Montross found herself surrounded by troubled teenagers dealing with extraordinary psychosocial stressors: poverty, trauma, family instability, mental illness [9, 10]. She watched them struggle. She wanted to help, but poetry and literature, as powerful as they were, felt insufficient. She began to wonder: what if she could do more?

The decision to pursue medicine came after lengthy soul-searching. Montross had never imagined herself as a doctor. She hadn't taken even a single pre-med course during her undergraduate years. But the pull was undeniable. She wanted to become a psychiatrist, to work with people in crisis, to understand the mind in ways that literature alone couldn't teach her [1, 9, 10]. So she enrolled in a post-baccalaureate program at Bryn Mawr College, spending a year taking all the prerequisite courses she'd skipped; organic chemistry, physics, biology. It was, she would later admit, painful [9, 10]. Science classes for a poet who'd spent years analyzing Rimbaud and crafting sestinas. But she persevered, and in September 2001, at the age of 28, Christine Montross began medical school at Brown University [1, 5, 7].

I think about what it means to start medical school at 28, when many students are fresh from undergraduate programs at 22 or 23. Montross brought with her a decade of adult life; a completed graduate degree, a teaching career, a marriage, published work. She had already established herself as a writer. She knew who she was in ways that younger students might not. And yet she chose to become, once again, a beginner. To sit in classrooms taking notes on glycolysis and the Krebs cycle. To memorize the brachial plexus and the branches of the aorta. To, in the very first year, walk into the anatomy lab and confront what every medical student must confront: a human body, in death, waiting to be dissected.

It was during that first year at Brown that Montross began writing what would become her first book [9, 10]. Immediately after beginning the process of dissecting a human body in anatomy lab, she knew the experience was rich to explore in written form. The fascination with the body had reemerged, accompanied by manifold emotions: the experience was simultaneously difficult, intimate, destructive, instructive, revelatory, and wild. She and her three lab partners were assigned a cadaver—a woman—whose hands, head, and feet were covered in cloth and tied in plastic, an attempt to depersonalize the body. And yet they felt compelled to name her. They called her Eve [1, 11].

"Body of Work: Meditations on Mortality from the Human Anatomy Lab," published in 2007 while Montross was in her final year at Brown, is structured around the dissection of Eve [11]. Each chapter corresponds to a different region of the body, from the chest to the head, tracing the meticulous process of exploration. But the book is far more than an anatomy text. It is a meditation on mortality, a philosophical inquiry into what it means to cut apart what was once alive, what was once a person with a life and a history and people who loved her. Montross writes with the precision of a scientist and the lyricism of a poet. She describes the physical reality of dissection—the smell, the texture, the difficulty of cutting through skin that has been preserved in formaldehyde—but she also delves into the psychological and emotional landscape of becoming a doctor.

The book grapples with questions that medical education rarely addresses explicitly: How do you maintain empathy while becoming inured to suffering? How do you touch a patient's body without embarrassment or violation of their privacy? How do you find the midpoint between excessive emotional involvement and complete lack of empathy: what medical educators call "detached concern," a phrase that itself contains a paradox? As Montross writes: "The midpoint in medicine between excessive emotional involvement with patients and a complete lack of empathy is not a simple one to locate. The former leads to exhaustion and burnout in the care provider; the latter gives rise to the all-too-familiar doctor with 'bad bedside manner,' whose patients feel unheard, uncared about, and, as a result, unsafe [11]."

She describes the shame she felt after the penis dissection, not because of puritanical attitudes toward genitals but because of inadequacy; the awareness that patients' comfort levels are often direct reflections of their physicians' comfort [11]. A gynecologist who addresses issues without embarrassment instantly puts patients at ease; a cardiologist who blushes when a patient opens her shirt creates discomfort. Montross wanted to be the former but found herself, in those early days, sometimes being the latter. The anatomy lab became a training ground not just for learning the parts of the body but for learning how to be at ease with bodies, including their most intimate parts.

But even beyond the practical question of comfort, there's the deeper philosophical problem: How do you allow yourself to feel the fullness of human emotion—the disgust, the faintness, the upset at seeing suffering—while simultaneously managing those feelings so you can provide care? "As medical students we are in the interspace between doctor and nondoctor," Montross writes. "We have the spontaneous feelings that nondoctors do when we are first exposed to sickness and injury. We feel upset and disgusted, and faint. Because we are in the interspace, however, we are aware that we must begin to manage those feelings and that, just as we must not blush when a woman opens her blouse nor cry when helping a family make decisions about a loved one's care, we must also touch and carry on conversations with patients who have seeping wounds, contagious rashes, disfiguring burns, bizarre delusions [11]."

The book also travels beyond the anatomy lab at Brown. Montross went to Padua, Italy, to see where Andreas Vesalius performed his historic dissections; illustrations from Vesalius's *De humani corporis fabrica* introduce each chapter of her book [9]. She went to Bologna to see the collection of wax anatomical sculptures used for teaching in the eighteenth century. She researched the history of cadaver procurement, from the Scottish "resurrectionists" Burke and Hare, who descended from grave robbing to murder to provide medical students with fresh bodies, to the complicated ethics of modern anatomical donation [11]. She situates her personal experience within centuries of medical history, showing how the practice of dissection has always existed at the intersection of science, ethics, religion, and law.

"Body of Work" was named an Editors' Choice by The New York Times and one of The Washington Post's best nonfiction books of 2007 [1, 7]. Rachel Hartigan Shea of The Washington Post called it "a beautiful book" that "offers a glimpse of a place off limits to anyone without Montross's clearsighted courage [12]." Kirkus Reviews noted it was "not for the squeamish, but an eye-opener for would-be doctors [13]." The book resonated with medical students and physicians who recognized their own experiences in Montross's words, and with general readers fascinated by the hidden world of medical training. Dr. Christine Montross appeared on C-SPAN's Q&A for an interview with Brian Lamb about the book, bringing her insights to a national audience [14].

After receiving her MD degree in 2006 and her Master of Medical Science degree in 2007, Dr. Montross completed her psychiatry residency at Brown in 2010 [1, 7]. During residency, she received the Isaac Ray Award in Psychiatry and the Martin B. Keller Outstanding Brown Psychiatry Resident Award [1, 7, 15]. She went on to become an assistant professor (later associate professor) of psychiatry and human behavior at the Warren Alpert Medical School of Brown University [15]. She also became a staff psychiatrist at Butler Hospital in Providence, Rhode Island, where she works on locked inpatient wards treating patients in acute psychiatric crisis [1, 10]. Additionally, she performs forensic psychiatric examinations; evaluations for legal proceedings, assessing competency to stand trial, criminal responsibility, risk of future violence [1, 7].

In 2010, Dr. Montross received the MacColl Johnson Fellowship in Poetry. She used the award money to conduct research in Paris on the origins of psychiatric treatment and to begin work on a collection of poetry, tentatively titled "Lunacy and Light [7, 15]." But as she worked, the project evolved. The poems transformed into prose, and what emerged was her second book: "Falling Into the Fire: A Psychiatrist's Encounters with the Mind in Crisis," published in 2014 [1, 16].

"Falling Into the Fire" is structured around case studies of psychiatric patients Dr. Montross treated during rounds at the locked inpatient ward [16]. The cases are extraordinary, almost unbelievable in their extremity. A young woman who habitually commits self-injury, ingesting light bulbs, a box of nails, zippers, and a steak knife. A new mother admitted with incessant visions of hurting her infant, so terrified of what she might do that she hid all the knives in her house. A recent college graduate, dressed in a tunic and declaring that love emanates from everything around him, brought to the ER by his alarmed girlfriend: is it ecstasy or psychosis? A man who keeps tearing at his skin and hair, spending thousands on treatments to correct his perceived "ugliness," suffering from severe body dysmorphic disorder. A woman so skilled at feigning epileptic seizures that staff feared she might actually die from status epilepticus [16].

Dr. Montross writes of these encounters with dramatic flair, ever empathetic but unsparing of her own negative feelings, fears, and frustrations. She's honest about the challenges: Diagnosis is not always easy. Even when a patient's backstory reveals plausible causes of illness, there's little therapy can do if the patient is unwilling to engage in treatment. Insurance limitations force discharge once patients are "stabilized," even when they clearly need longer care. The woman who repeatedly swallows dangerous objects incites frustration in staff who feel helpless to stop the cycle. Dr. Montross examines how emotion can interfere with proper care, how the repeated admission of the same patient for self-destructive behaviors can lead to staff burnout and diminished empathy.

The book also explores strange paradoxes in psychiatric care. Patients afflicted with extreme forms of body dissatisfaction—people who want a healthy limb amputated, for instance—are sometimes "cured" if the surgery actually takes place, which raises troubling questions about the nature of psychiatric illness and the ethics of treatment. Is it appropriate to amputate a healthy limb if that's what will relieve the patient's suffering? Or is such an action a violation of medical ethics? These are the kinds of impossible questions Dr. Montross grapples with daily in her practice [16].

Throughout the book, Dr. Montross interweaves anecdotes from her domestic life with her wife, Deborah Salem Smith, and their two young children [8]. She reflects on her own fortune, her relatively stable mental health, and her ability to function in the world. There's an awareness, threading through every chapter, that mental illness could happen to anyone. As she writes in one of the book's most powerful passages: "Standing on the edge with my patients—abiding with them—means that I must harbor a true awareness that I, too, could lose my child through the play of circumstance over which I have no control. I could lose my home, my financial security, my safety. I could lose my mind. Any of us could [16]." This awareness of shared vulnerability, this refusal to see psychiatric patients as fundamentally different from herself, defines Dr. Montross's approach to psychiatry. Mental illness is not a moral failing or a character flaw. It's a biological reality that can strike anyone, often without warning, sometimes without obvious cause.

The book was named a New Yorker Book to Watch Out For [1, 7]. Reviews praised Dr. Montross's ability to present unique patient histories with an insightful mind constantly searching for new means of treatment, her integration of historical research with contemporary case studies. The New Yorker noted that "Montross explores the practical, emotional, and philosophical challenges of working with patients whose illnesses of the mind are often intractable and deeply disturbing [17]." Shelf Awareness called it "pragmatic and compassionate," noting that Dr. Montross is "empathetic and informative" in her "fascinating look into the convoluted world of psychiatry and mental illness [17]." But not all responses were positive. Some readers, particularly those with mental illness, found parts of the book troubling. Dr. Montross writes about playing a game with other doctors and nurses on the ward; looking at patient photos and trying to guess their diagnoses based on appearance [16]. She acknowledges this wasn't a particularly sensitive practice, but some readers found it deeply offensive, a reminder of how even well-meaning clinicians can objectify patients in moments of stress or boredom.

This criticism points to a tension in physician-memoir writing: How honest should doctors be about their own failings, their own moments of insensitivity or burnout? Is it better to present an idealized version of medical practice, hiding the messy reality? Or is it more valuable to show the truth, even when that truth is uncomfortable? Dr. Montross chose honesty, and while that opened her to criticism, it also made her work more real, more useful to other clinicians who recognize their own struggles in her words.

In 2015, Dr. Montross was awarded a Guggenheim Fellowship in General Nonfiction, one of the most prestigious honors a writer can receive [6, 18]. She used the fellowship to research her third book, initially titled "Acquainted With the Night" but ultimately published in 2020 as "Waiting for an Echo: The Madness of American Incarceration [19]." The book investigates what happens to people with serious mental illness when they end up in the American criminal justice system instead of in psychiatric hospitals, which, increasingly, is where they end up.

Dr. Montross spent years researching correctional institutions both in the United States and abroad. She visited the Cook County Jail in Chicago, one of the largest jails in the country, where thousands of inmates with mental illness are housed in conditions that can only be described as inhumane. She studied Halden Prison in Norway, often called the most humane prison in the world, where the recidivism rate is dramatically lower than in American prisons because rehabilitation is prioritized over punishment. She interviewed inmates, corrections officers, lawyers, judges, mental health professionals. She examined sentencing practices that routinely reach decades into the future, that impose life sentences or even multiple consecutive life sentences. She asked: What is the purpose of this extreme sentencing? To deter crime? To keep society safe? To exact revenge? And which of these goals, whether stated or unstated, are actually being met? [5, 20].

What Dr. Montross discovered was horrifying. The deinstitutionalization of psychiatric hospitals in the 1960s and 1970s, intended to free patients from abusive conditions, but had the consequence of shifting large numbers of mentally ill people from therapeutic settings into punitive ones. Jails and prisons became, by default, the largest mental health treatment facilities in America, while they were never designed for that purpose. When the treating facility is a prison, Dr. Montross writes, "safety, security and punishment necessarily take precedence over recovery and care [19]." Mentally ill inmates often can't follow prison rules because their illness prevents them from doing so. They're punished for behaviors that are symptoms of their disease. Solitary confinement, one of the most common punishments, is particularly devastating for people with mental illness, often causing or exacerbating psychosis, depression, anxiety, suicidal ideation.

The book is divided into three sections: "Our Prisoners," "Our Prisons," and "Our Choice." The first section explains why so many obviously mentally ill women and men end up in prison; most crimes they commit are caused, at least in part, by their mental illness, and police, attorneys, and judges are often ill-equipped to recognize psychiatric crises or to divert people toward treatment instead of incarceration. The second section includes chilling case studies of ineffective incarceration, particularly regarding solitary confinement, showing the deep psychological damage inflicted by the nation's punitive structures. The third section offers hope, chronicling Dr. Montross's research in Norway and other countries where prisons have drastically lowered recidivism rates by emphasizing human rehabilitation over revenge [19].

Dr. Montross concludes by quoting James Baldwin: "Nothing can be changed until it is faced." In this revelatory book, she faces the problem head-on. She demonstrates that everybody in American society—the imprisoned mentally ill, the rest of the prison population, prison staff, police, attorneys, judges, jurors, loved ones of inmates, residents of neighborhoods where former inmates are released, taxpayers whose money funds punishment instead of rehabilitation—experiences harm from the status quo. The system helps no one. It brutalizes everyone it touches.

"Waiting for an Echo" was named a New York Times Book to Watch For, a Time Magazine Book to Read, an Amazon.com Best Book of the Month, and a finalist for the Los Angeles Times Book Prize. The New York Times Book Review called it "a haunting and harrowing indictment…a significant achievement." Kirkus Reviews praised it as a revelatory book where "the author faces the problem head-on." Susannah Cahalan, author of "Brain on Fire," wrote: "Christine Montross, a psychiatrist, writes from inside the ranks of our broken mental health system, but she does so with a poet's eye, bringing to life the human toll behind the horrifying statistics. The result is a rallying cry that is both personal and universal, and, hopefully, one that we will not be able to ignore" [1, 19, 21, 22].

Throughout her career, Dr. Montross has written for numerous national publications including The New York Times, The New England Journal of Medicine, The Washington Post Book World, Good Housekeeping, and O, The Oprah Magazine. She has continued to publish poetry in literary journals [1]. Her manuscript "Embouchure" was a finalist for the National Poetry Series. In addition to her Guggenheim Fellowship, she has been named a 2017–2018 Faculty Fellow at the Cogut Center for the Humanities and was awarded the 2009 Eugene and Marilyn Glick Emerging Indiana Authors Award [1, 7, 15].

As an educator, Dr. Montross serves as co-director of the Medical Humanities and Bioethics Scholarly Concentration at Brown's medical school [1, 15]. She teaches future physicians not just how to diagnose and treat, but how to think ethically, how to consider the larger social contexts of illness, how to maintain their humanity in a profession that can be dehumanizing. She brings her background in literature and poetry into medical education, showing students that the skills of close reading, of attention to language, of empathy and imagination, are essential to good doctoring.

Dr. Montross asks, "How do we find the midpoint between excessive emotional involvement and complete lack of empathy?" This question isn't just about anatomy lab or bedside manner. It's the central question of being a physician-writer. How do you write about patients without exploiting their suffering for your own literary purposes? How do you tell true stories while protecting privacy? How do you reveal your own doubts and failures without undermining patients' trust? Dr. Montross navigates these tensions thoughtfully, changing details to preserve confidentiality, seeking permissions where possible, always asking: am I honoring these stories or am I using them?

Her work reminds us why we need more physician-writers, especially in psychiatry. Mental illness remains stigmatized, misunderstood, feared. Psychiatric patients are often portrayed in media as violent, dangerous, unpredictable; when the reality is that people with mental illness are far more likely to be victims of violence than perpetrators. By writing about her patients with empathy and nuance, by showing their humanity alongside their symptoms, Dr. Montross challenges those stereotypes. By writing about the criminalization of mental illness, she forces us to confront a system that punishes people for being sick. By writing honestly about her own struggles with maintaining detached concern, she normalizes the emotional labor of psychiatric care.

And her work also reminds us why medical education requires the humanities. The technical knowledge of medicine—the anatomy, the pharmacology, the diagnostic criteria—is necessary but insufficient. Physicians also need to understand ethics, history, literature, and philosophy. They need to know how to listen to stories, how to interpret narratives, and how to communicate with empathy. They need to grapple with questions that have no clear answers: What is a good life? What is a good death? When should we intervene and when should we allow suffering to run its course? What do we owe to each other? What does it mean to be human?

These are questions that anatomy textbooks don't answer, that clinical practice guidelines don't address. But they're questions that every physician confronts daily. Dr. Montross brings the tools of literature and poetry to these questions, showing how the humanities aren't decoration or distraction from medicine; they're essential to it.

References

1. Montross C. Christine Montross [Official website]. n.d. https://christinemontross.com/.
2. Basketball Reference. Eric Montross. n.d. https://www.basketball-reference.com/players/m/montrer01.html.
3. CBS News. Eric Montross, former UNC basketball star and NBA big man, dies at 52. 2023, December 18. https://www.cbsnews.com/news/eric-montross-dies-unc-basketball-star-dead-age-52-cause-of-death-cancer/.
4. Penguin Random House. Christine Montross [Author page]. n.d. https://www.penguinrandomhouse.com/authors/230433/christine-montross/.
5. Klein JM. The madness of prison. University of Michigan Alumni Association; 2020, August 6. https://alumni.umich.edu/michigan-alum/the-madness-of-prison/.
6. John Simon Guggenheim Memorial Foundation. Christine Montross. 2015. https://www.gf.org/fellows/christine-montross/.
7. Amazon. Christine Montross: Books, biography, latest update. n.d. https://www.amazon.com/stores/author/B001JPC0L2/about?ccs_id=b1b451ac-9f2e-44c6-9761-3c1dee528201.
8. Goodman L. Alumni profile: Deborah Salem Smith '96, a playwright who probes gray areas. Princeton Alumni Weekly. 2012, April 25. https://paw.princeton.edu/article/alumni-profile-deborah-salem-smith-96-playwright-who-probes-gray-areas.
9. Harvey CB. Anatomy lesson. Brown Alumni Magazine. 2007, September 26. https://www.brownalumnimagazine.com/articles/2007-09-26/anatomy-lesson.

10. In-House Staff & Duan C. Physician-author series: Christine Montross. In-House. 2015, December 15. https://in-housestaff.org/physicians-writers-christine-montross-123.
11. Montross C. Body of work: meditations on mortality from the human anatomy lab. New York: Penguin Books; 2007.
12. Shea RH. Anatomy of an education. The Washington Post. 2007, July 16. https://www.washingtonpost.com/archive/style/2007/07/17/anatomy-of-an-education/1df87d9c-2521-4d05-a2ef-cf25d222f58c/.
13. Kirkus Reviews. Body of work: Meditations on mortality from the human anatomy lab. 2007, June 25. https://www.kirkusreviews.com/book-reviews/christine-montross/body-of-work/.
14. C-SPAN. Christine Montross [Video]. 2007, July 12. https://www.c-span.org/program/qa/christine-montross/178717.
15. Brown University. Christine E Montross: Associate Professor of Psychiatry and Human Behavior, Associate Professor of Medical Science. n.d. https://vivo.brown.edu/display/cmontros.
16. Montross C. Falling into the fire: a psychiatrist's encounters with the mind in crisis. New York, NY: Penguin; 2014.
17. Montross C. Falling into the fire. New York: Penguin Press; 2013. https://www.amazon.com/Falling-Into-Fire-Psychiatrists-Encounters/dp/1594203938.
18. Orenstein D. Two professors win Guggenheim fellowships. Brown University; 2015. https://archive2.news.brown.edu/2007-2015/articles/2015/04/guggenheims.html.
19. Montross C. Waiting for an echo: the madness of American incarceration. New York: Penguin Books; 2020.
20. Davies D. Psychiatrist: America's "extremely punitive" prisons make mental illness worse. NPR. 2020, July 16 https://www.npr.org/sections/health-shots/2020/07/16/891438605/psychiatrist-americas-extremely-punitive-prisons-make-mental-illness-worse.
21. Kirkus Reviews. Waiting for an echo: the madness of American incarceration. 2020. https://www.kirkusreviews.com/book-reviews/christine-montross/waiting-for-an-echo/.
22. BookBrowse. Waiting for an echo: the madness of American incarceration [Review] 2020. https://www.bookbrowse.com/reviews/index.cfm/book_number/4134/waiting-for-an-echo#media_reviews.

Chapter 12
Rachel Naomi Remen, MD

One curious aspect of entering a world of chronic disease, as a patient, was encountering its many biases within medicine, even amongst those who inherently mean well. Some conditions are colored with a brush of pity and sympathy, while others are given a tint of scorn. Even excluding the influence of societal biases surrounding race, ethnicity, language, religion and gender, simply having that ICD code recorded in a chart unlocks sentiments within physicians which patients are then tasked to modify. Many diagnoses are well delineated in the medical texts, but even more still carry questions as to their pathophysiology and presentation in different patients. And outside of the medical community, particularly amongst women, diagnoses that are so prevalent, they may as well be considered "common," are held in secret with a sense of shame, revealing themselves only in anonymous online chat rooms. Dr. Rachel Remen explores these biases we all hold, while touching the specific solution to many of the angst: listening. And not the exercise that is in preparation for rebuttal but listening to understand. Our similarities in sickness and in health, she illuminates beautifully, and I am honored to share her work with you.

I discovered Dr. Remen's work during my pediatric residency, at a time when I was struggling with the emotional weight of caring for critically ill children while managing my own chronic illness. Someone had left a dog-eared copy of Kitchen Table Wisdom in the residents' lounge, its spine cracked at multiple places, evidence of many hands seeking solace in its pages. I picked it up during a particularly difficult night shift, after losing a patient I had grown attached to over months of hospitalizations. The first story I read was about a woman with cancer who had been told she was dying, but who chose to live fully in whatever time remained. Dr. Remen wrote about how this patient taught her that healing and curing are not the same thing; that wholeness can exist even in the presence of disease.

That distinction lodged itself in my chest like a seed waiting for the right conditions to germinate. As someone who had spent years trying to "fix" my own incurable condition, the idea that I might already be whole felt both revolutionary and deeply threatening. If I was already whole, what had I been striving toward all these

O. M. Cox, *The Pen, The Stethoscope, and The Scalpel*,
https://doi.org/10.1007/978-3-032-19406-0_12

years? And yet, there was something profoundly liberating in the possibility that my value as a person—and as a physician—was not contingent on achieving perfect health, either for myself or for my patients.

Dr. Rachel Naomi Remen was born on February 8, 1938, in New York City, into a family steeped in Jewish intellectual and spiritual tradition [1, 2]. Her grandfather, an orthodox rabbi and scholar of the Kabbalah, would become one of the most formative influences in her life and work [2, 3]. From him, she learned to see the world as a web of connection, to understand that blessing one another is what fills our emptiness and heals our loneliness. These early lessons in seeing the sacred in the everyday would later inform her revolutionary approach to medicine, though she could not have known it as a child listening to her grandfather's stories at the kitchen table.

Dr. Remen attended Cornell Medical School, graduating in 1962 at a time when women physicians were rare enough to be remarkable [4, 5]. The medical culture of that era was even more brutally focused on objectivity and emotional distance than it is today. Students were taught to see disease, not people; to value knowledge above wisdom; to cure at all costs. Dr. Remen excelled in this environment, completing her internship and residency in pediatrics at New York Hospital (1962–1965), followed by a fellowship at Stanford University School of Medicine (1965–1967) [1]. She became an assistant professor of pediatrics at Stanford (1967–1974) and eventually Associate Director of the Pediatrics Clinic at Stanford Medical School [1, 4]. By all external measures, she was succeeding brilliantly in her chosen field.

But there was a shadow accompanying her success, a secret she carried through medical school and into her early years of practice. At age 15, Dr. Remen was diagnosed with Crohn's disease, a chronic inflammatory bowel condition that would require her to undergo major surgery seven times over the course of her life [5, 6]. She has now lived with this disease for over 70 years, navigating the medical system from both sides of the stethoscope [2]. This dual perspective—physician and patient, healer and wounded—would ultimately become the wellspring of her most important contributions to medicine and literature.

In the 1970s, Dr. Remen encountered the Esalen Institute and its pioneering work in humanistic psychology and holistic health. This meeting proved transformative. She found herself drawn to a radically different vision of medicine, one that honored the whole person—body, mind, and spirit—rather than reducing patients to their pathology. She became one of the earliest pioneers in the mind/body holistic health movement and the first to recognize the role of the spirit in health and the recovery from illness [7, 8]. It was a vision that resonated with what she had experienced as a patient: the loneliness of being seen only as a disease process, the yearning to be met as a full human being in all one's complexity and vulnerability.

Making the decision to leave her prestigious position at Stanford to pursue this new direction required tremendous courage. She was abandoning the traditional academic medicine career path she had worked so hard to achieve. She risked being dismissed by colleagues as having gone "soft," as pursuing something less rigorous, less scientific, less legitimate. But Dr. Remen had learned something crucial through her own experiences with chronic illness: that the things we cannot measure may be the things that ultimately sustain and enrich our lives. She chose to follow that wisdom, even when it meant stepping away from conventional success.

In 1980, Dr. Remen published her first book, "Human Patient," one of the earliest books on holistic medicine and the medicine of the whole person [4, 9]. The book called on both the medical profession and patients to become aware of untapped strengths and human capacities; qualities such as courage, wisdom, humor, creativity, compassion, and imagination. This pioneering work laid the groundwork for her later contributions to integrative medicine and relationship-centered care [6].

In 1986, Dr. Remen co-founded the Commonweal Cancer Help Program in Bolinas, California, with Michael Lerner [4, 7, 10]. This week-long retreat program for people with cancer was revolutionary in its approach, focusing not on curing disease but on helping participants reclaim a sense of wholeness and meaning in their lives [7, 8]. The program was featured in Bill Moyers' acclaimed PBS series Healing and the Mind, bringing Dr. Remen's work to national attention [7]. For nearly three decades, she would care for thousands of people with cancer and their families, sitting with them in their darkest moments, witnessing their courage, and learning from their wisdom.

But Dr. Remen's most far-reaching contribution to medicine came through medical education. She recognized that physicians themselves were suffering; from burnout, from cynicism, from a loss of meaning in their work. The same system that failed to see patients as whole people was also dehumanizing the doctors trying to care for them. In 1991, she founded what would later become the Remen Institute for the Study of Health and Illness (RISHI) , a training institute for health professionals seeking to practice medicine with greater compassion, meaning, and connection [7].

At UCSF School of Medicine, Dr. Remen developed an elective course called "The Healer's Art," an innovative discovery model course in values clarification and professionalism for medical students [6, 7]. In a medical education landscape dominated by biochemistry, pathophysiology, and clinical skills, this course dared to ask students to reflect on what it means to be a healer, to examine their own mortality and vulnerability, to explore the spiritual dimensions of caring for the sick. The course used storytelling, small group discussions, and contemplative practices to help students reconnect with the idealism and compassion that had drawn them to medicine in the first place [6, 7].

The Healer's Art was so successful at UCSF that other medical schools began requesting permission to adopt it. Today, this groundbreaking curriculum is taught at more than 90 American medical schools and in seven countries abroad [6, 11]. Schools like Yale, Harvard, Brown, Stanford, and Dartmouth have integrated Dr. Remen's approach into their training of future physicians. US News & World Report has called it "a profoundly innovative curriculum on reintegrating the heart and soul into contemporary medicine and restoring medicine to its integrity as a calling and a work of healing [11]."

What makes The Healer's Art so powerful is that it addresses something most medical education ignores: the interior life of the physician. It acknowledges that doctors are human beings who will face loss, failure, and their own mortality. It teaches that our wounds, rather than being sources of shame to be hidden, can become sources of compassion and connection. Dr. Remen often quotes the concept of the "wounded healer," the idea that we can serve others precisely because we understand suffering from the inside. This was not abstract theory for her; it was lived experience. Her Crohn's disease, with all its limitation, had taught her things about healing that no textbook could convey.

Throughout her career as a medical educator and therapist, Dr. Remen was also writing. She kept notebooks filled with stories from her patients, stories that illuminated the mystery and power of the human spirit in the face of illness and loss. These were not case studies in the traditional medical sense, with their emphasis on symptoms, diagnosis, and treatment outcomes. They were narratives that honored the full complexity of human experience, that found meaning in suffering without minimizing its reality, that witnessed transformation without prescribing it [6].

In 1996, Dr. Remen published her second book, "Kitchen Table Wisdom: Stories That Heal" which became an immediate New York Times bestseller [6, 12]. The book is a collection of true stories drawn from Dr. Remen's decades of work with patients facing cancer and other serious illnesses. Each story is short—often just a few pages—but together they create a tapestry that reveals fundamental truths about human nature, about suffering and healing, about connection and isolation, about the difference between curing and healing.

The book's title evokes the oral tradition of wisdom-sharing that happens around kitchen tables, where people speak from the heart about what matters most. Dr. Remen wrote in her introduction: "Despite the awesome powers of technology, many of us still do not live very well. We may need to listen to one another's stories again [12]." This simple observation captured something many readers recognized immediately; a hunger for authentic human connection, for stories that acknowledged life's difficulties without offering false comfort, for wisdom that came not from experts but from ordinary people facing extraordinary circumstances.

"Kitchen Table Wisdom" has now sold millions of copies and been translated into 23 languages. It won the 1996 Wilbur Award for best work of spiritual nonfiction and the 2000 Friends of Libraries USA Readers' Choice Award. More significantly, it has been adopted as a textbook in numerous nursing and medical schools, introducing generations of healthcare students to a different way of thinking about their work [6, 13]. The book demonstrated that rigorous medicine and deep humanity are not opposites but necessary partners in the work of healing.

The success of "Kitchen Table Wisdom," established Dr. Remen as a master storyteller whose work transcended the typical boundaries between medical literature, spiritual writing, and popular psychology. Her stories worked on multiple levels; they were moving and beautifully written, they offered practical wisdom for living, and they subtly challenged readers to reconsider their assumptions about illness, health, and what it means to live a meaningful life.

In 2000, Dr. Remen published her second major bestseller, "My Grandfather's Blessings: Stories of Strength, Refuge and Belonging [14]." This national bestseller, published in 21 languages, drew directly on the wisdom she had learned from her grandfather, the Orthodox rabbi who taught her to see life as a web of connection [6,

14]. The book's central message—that blessing one another fills our emptiness and heals our loneliness—spoke to a deep human need for belonging and sacred connection. Through stories from her patients and her own life, Dr. Remen showed how we might recognize and receive the blessings that life offers us, even in dark times.

She also published "The Will to Live and Other Mysteries," in 2001, a collection that probed deeper into the experience of mystery and its power to transform our lives [15]. The book challenged our cultural worship of science by acknowledging that, despite all our medical advances, we still cannot fully explain how healing happens. Dr. Remen shared compelling stories of people who, against all odds, embodied the will to live and opened to the power of mystery as a healing resource.

More recently, Dr. Remen wrote "The Birthday of the World," a children's book that retells a Kabbalistic story about finding light in the darkness, one spark at a time [16]. Even in this work for younger readers, her essential message remained consistent: that we are all here to find the light and change the world, that connection is what matters most, that everyone has gifts to offer.

The literary impact of Dr. Remen's work extends far beyond sales figures and translations, impressive as those are. She helped bolster the genre of "narrative medicine" or "medical humanities," writing that bridges the worlds of clinical medicine and human storytelling. Her books demonstrated that medical experiences could be sources of profound literary and spiritual insight, that the stories emerging from illness and healing deserved to be told with the same care and artistry as any other significant human experience. Her influence can be seen in the work of other physician-writers who have followed, from Dr. Atul Gawande to Dr. Paul Kalanithi, and to countless others who write about medicine in ways that honor both scientific rigor and human complexity. She showed that doctors need not choose between their scientific training and their capacity for wonder, between professional competence and personal vulnerability, between helping and being helped.

Dr. Remen's books have also had a significant impact on popular culture beyond the medical community. They have been embraced by readers dealing with illness, yes, but also by anyone grappling with loss, transition, or the search for meaning. Her work has influenced the field of positive psychology, the mindfulness movement in healthcare, and the growing interest in spiritual but not religious approaches to life's big questions [6]. Deepak Chopra has called her "a pioneer in the medicine of the future," while Bernie Siegel praised "Kitchen Table Wisdom," as "a beautiful book about life, the only true teacher [12]."

In recognition of her contributions to medicine and medical education, Dr. Remen has received numerous honors, including three honorary degrees. She received the prestigious Bravewell Award as one of the earliest pioneers of Integrative Medicine and Relationship-Centered Care [6, 17]. In 2013, the UCSF School of Medicine awarded her the Gold-Headed Cane, given to someone who exemplifies and teaches the qualities and values of the true physician [6]. These awards acknowledged what her students and readers already knew: that Dr. Remen had helped create a new paradigm in medicine, one that could hold both scientific excellence and human wisdom, both technical skill and compassionate presence.

Today, at 87 years old, Dr. Remen continues her work. She is Clinical Professor Emeritus of Family and Community Medicine at UCSF School of Medicine and Professor of Family Medicine at Wright State University Boonshoft School of Medicine in Ohio, where the Remen Institute relocated in 2016 [6]. She continues to train health professionals in relationship-centered care and to speak and write about the integration of compassion, meaning, and service in healthcare. Most recently, she appeared on a podcast with Surgeon General Vivek Murthy, her former student, discussing the journey to becoming a healer; evidence that her influence continues to shape medicine at the highest levels [18].

Dr. Remen's seven-decade experience with Crohn's disease has been central to her work, providing her with the insider's perspective that makes her writing so authentic and her teaching so powerful. She has written openly about the many surgeries, the pain, the restrictions, and also about what chronic illness has taught her [6]. In her work, she has never presented herself as someone who has transcended suffering or achieved some special enlightenment. Instead, she writes as a fellow traveler, someone who knows the territory of illness from the inside and can therefore be a trustworthy guide for others navigating similar terrain.

Her concept of "kitchen table wisdom" itself represents a challenge to medical hierarchy. It suggests that the most important knowledge doesn't flow only from experts to patients, from doctors to the sick, but circulates among all of us who are living everyday human lives. It acknowledges that patients have wisdom to share with their doctors, that suffering can be a teacher, that the very experiences we're taught to fear and avoid—illness, loss, mortality—can open us to deeper understanding and more authentic connection.

This practice of remembering our common humanity seems simple, almost obvious. And yet it is profoundly countercultural in a medical system that emphasizes expertise, hierarchy, and emotional distance. Dr. Remen's great gift has been to show us, through her stories and her teaching, that we need not choose between competence and compassion, between scientific rigor and human warmth. The best medicine, she demonstrates, includes both, or rather, recognizes them as inseparable. In a world that too often reduces people to their diagnoses, their problems, their needs, Dr. Remen invites us to see and be seen more fully.

References

1. Prabook World Biographical Encyclopedia. Rachel Naomi Remen. n.d. https://prabook.com/web/rachel_naomi.remen/3500818.
2. The On Being Project. Rachel Naomi Remen—how we live with loss [Interview with Krista Tippett]. n.d. https://onbeing.org/programs/rachel-naomi-remen-how-we-live-with-loss/.
3. Remen RN. My grandfather's blessings: stories of strength, refuge, and belonging. New York: Riverhead Books; 2000.
4. YWCA Golden Gate Silicon Valley. Rachel Naomi Remen, M.D. [2005 Health & Medicine Honoree]. 2005. https://yourywca.org/honorees/rachel-naomi-remen-m-d/.

5. National Library of Medicine. Changing the face of medicine: Rachel Naomi Remen. n.d. https://cfmedicine.nlm.nih.gov/physicians/biography_264.html.
6. Remen RN. Rachel Naomi Remen, MD [Official website]. n.d. https://www.rachelremen.com/.
7. Remen Institute for the Study of Health and Illness (RISHI). Home. n.d. https://rishiprograms.org/.
8. The New School at Commonweal. Rachel Naomi Remen, MD. n.d. https://tns.commonweal.org/podcasts/rachel-naomi-remen-md/.
9. Remen RN. The human patient. Anchor Books; 1980. https://www.goodreads.com/book/show/461724.Human_Patient.
10. Healing Circles Global. Starting Commonweal and Healing Circles. n.d. https://healingcircles-global.org/starting-commonweal-and-healing-circles/.
11. Wright State University Newsroom. Boonshoft School of Medicine welcomes the Remen Institute for the Study of Health and Illness. 2016, April 12. https://webapp2.wright.edu/web1/newsroom/2016/04/12/boonshoft-school-of-medicine-welcomes-the-remen-institute-for-the-study-of-health-and-illness/.
12. Remen RN. Kitchen table wisdom: stories that heal. Riverhead Books; 1996. https://www.amazon.com/Kitchen-Wisdom-Paperback-Rachel-Foreword/dp/0330363298.
13. Kirkus Reviews. Kitchen table wisdom. 1996. https://www.kirkusreviews.com/book-reviews/rachel-naomi-remen/kitchen-table-wisdom/.
14. Remen RN. My grandfather's blessings. Riverhead Books; 2000. https://www.penguinrandomhouse.com/books/348373/my-grandfathers-blessings-by-rachel-naomi-remen/.
15. Remen RN. The will to live and other mysteries [Audio recording]. Sounds True. 2001. https://www.goodreads.com/book/show/461701.The_Will_to_Live_and_Other_Mysteries.
16. Remen RN. The birthday of the world. Abrams Books for Young Readers; 2022. https://www.goodreads.com/book/show/60310820-the-birthday-of-the-world.
17. House Calls with Dr. Vivek Murthy. Dr. Rachel Naomi Remen: can we all be healers? [Audio podcast episode]. Apple Podcasts. 2023, September 5. https://podcasts.apple.com/us/podcast/dr-rachel-naomi-remen-can-we-all-be-healers/id1621592840?i=1000626877027.
18. House Calls with Dr. Vivek Murthy. Dr. Rachel Naomi Remen: Q&A on becoming a healer [Audio podcast episode]. Apple Podcasts. 2024, March 6. https://podcasts.apple.com/us/podcast/dr-rachel-naomi-remen-q-a-on-becoming-a-healer/id1621592840?i=1000648141194.

Chapter 13
Lydia Kang, MD

For most authors, fiction represents a sort of cataclysmic release from the confines of everyday, so much so that developing characters, building worlds, engineering conversations and scenes is an addictive exercise. That we have not completed multiple novels is often not due to insufficient imagination, but from the limitations of time. From a purely artistic perspective, I have viewed fictional prose as documenting scenes already playing within the mind. And to do so in as realistic a way as possible requires acute observation of the world, and a keen understanding of human tendencies. The best fictional authors must first appreciate the complexities of people to perfectly place them in any environment. How they grow, how they learn, how they love, and how they grieve. When combined with an understanding of physiology, evidence-based psychology and precise anatomy, the best sort of fiction, which we may all dive into, is created. We have all experienced the jolting moment when biologic impossibilities are allowed into stories and have all suspended disbelief at quixotical heroes whom we otherwise have come to appreciate. In Dr. Lydia Kang's work, these practices are unnecessary, as she demonstrates a critical understanding of what makes people and worlds tick. She is my favorite kind of physician-writer, who recognizes the value of good science in science fiction, and multi-dimensional personalities in narrative protagonists.

Dr. Lydia Kang was born on October 4, 1971, in Baltimore, Maryland, into a family that would nurture both her scientific curiosity and her creative spirit. Growing up in the Baltimore suburbs, she attended Roland Park Country School, an all-girls preparatory institution [1–4]. It was there, in the crucible of rigorous academics and encouraging mentorship, that young Lydia Kang discovered her dual passions: the precision of science and the boundless possibilities of storytelling [3, 4].

These two loves—seemingly divergent in the eyes of conventional wisdom—would eventually converge in ways that the teenage Kang could scarcely have imagined. An organic chemistry class at Roland Park Country School sparked ideas that would later bloom into novels. A haunting poem she read in elementary school

O. M. Cox, *The Pen, The Stethoscope, and The Scalpel*,
https://doi.org/10.1007/978-3-032-19406-0_13

planted seeds that would grow into entire fictional worlds. Rather than choosing between the laboratory and the library, she would ultimately claim both as her territory, refusing to accept the false dichotomy that so often pushes young people toward one path or another [1].

After graduating from Roland Park Country School in 1989, Dr. Kang pursued her undergraduate education at Columbia University in New York City, where she majored in biology with a premed focus while minoring in English [1, 2, 5]. This academic combination was telling; even then, she was building the foundation for a career that would require both scientific rigor and narrative artistry. During her undergraduate years and continuing into graduate school, she worked as a research assistant in Columbia's Department of Biology, gaining hands-on experience with the scientific method that would later inform her approach to both medicine and fiction writing [2].

Dr. Kang earned her MD from New York University's Grossman School of Medicine in 1998, entering a medical education system that, despite progress, still often separated the art from the science of healing [1, 5]. The late 1990s medical training environment emphasized evidence-based practice and technological advancement, but the humanities—the stories of patients, the narrative arc of illness, the literary dimensions of suffering—were frequently relegated to the margins of medical education.

She completed her Internal Medicine residency at NYU Langone Health's Bellevue Hospital, one of the oldest public hospitals in America and an institution legendary for training physicians in the realities of urban medicine [2, 6]. Bellevue, with its diverse patient population and its historical significance in American medical education, left an indelible mark on Dr. Kang. She would later describe how Bellevue's history seemed to seep into her consciousness, creating a fascination with medical history that would eventually manifest in her writing. When she read Deborah Blum's nonfiction book "The Poisoner's Handbook," which focused heavily on Bellevue and the birth of forensic medicine in New York City, she knew she had found her setting and time period for what would become some of her most acclaimed historical fiction [4].

From 2001 to 2002, Dr. Kang served as Chief Resident at NYU Langone, a position that recognized her clinical excellence and leadership abilities. Following her chief residency, she remained at NYU as an attending physician, where she founded the inpatient Palliative Care consultation service, a testament to her recognition that medicine must address not just biological disease but also suffering, meaning, and quality of life [2, 6]. This early work in palliative care demonstrated her commitment to seeing patients as whole people navigating difficult journeys, not merely as collections of symptoms requiring technical interventions.

In 2006, Dr. Kang made a significant geographical and professional move, relocating to Omaha, Nebraska, to join the University of Nebraska Medical Center as an Assistant Professor in the Division of General Internal Medicine [2]. Her husband, an oncologist, would join her in building both their medical careers and their family in the Midwest [2]. They would raise three children together while maintaining demanding professional lives; she in primary care internal medicine and writing, he in cancer treatment [2].

It was in Omaha, Dr. Kang has said, that she truly began writing in earnest. In 2009, she joined the Seven Doctors Project at UNMC—a writing workshop that pairs UNMC faculty members with local writers—initially wanting to write poetry and medical memoir essays [1, 2, 7–9]. By her own admission, the early attempts were "really horrible poetry, really bad stuff," but the creative exercise proved surprisingly enjoyable [7]. She attended writing seminars and produced what she calls "practice novels," the essential apprenticeship work that most successful authors complete before finding their voice and their audience [7, 8].

By 2010, Dr. Kang was ready to test a more developed idea: a young adult science fiction novel centered on a protagonist living with Ondine's curse, a rare condition (actually called congenital central hypoventilation syndrome) in which the automatic control of breathing is impaired, potentially causing respiratory arrest during sleep. This melding of genuine medical knowledge with speculative fiction would become Dr. Kang's signature approach; stories that respected biological reality even while pushing into imaginative territory [1, 10].

That novel, "Control," was published in 2013 as Dr. Kang's debut work of fiction. Set in the year 2150, "Control" follows Zelia, a young woman whose genetic modifications and rare condition make her a target in a dystopian future where genetic "perfection" is valued above all else. The novel garnered praise for its scientific plausibility, its breakneck pacing, and its exploration of what it means to be human in a world increasingly capable of engineering humanity itself. James Dashner, author of "The Maze Runner," called it a "thrilling ride," while readers compared it favorably to classics of young adult dystopian fiction like "Uglies [10]."

A sequel, "Catalyst," followed in 2015, continuing Zelia's story as she and her fellow genetic "outcasts" struggle to find acceptance in a society that views their mutations with fear and disgust [11]. The themes resonating through both books—the value of human diversity, the ethics of genetic engineering, the tension between scientific progress and human dignity—reflected Dr. Kang's deep engagement with the moral questions that medicine continually poses.

But Dr. Kang's creative ambitions extended beyond her Control series. In 2016, she published "The November Girl, " a haunting young adult novel set on Isle Royale in Lake Superior. The book won the 2018 Nebraska Book Award for Young Adult Literature, establishing Dr. Kang as a significant voice in contemporary YA fiction [1, 12]. The novel tells the story of a girl with violence running through her veins who meets a boy fleeing an abusive home; a premise that allowed Dr. Kang to explore trauma, connection, and the wild power of nature through a supernatural lens.

In 2018, Dr. Kang published "Toxic," a young adult space opera about a genetically created teenage girl abandoned on a biological spaceship, and the mercenary boy doomed to die there [13]. The novel won the YARWA Athena Award for speculative fiction and was selected as a Junior Library Guild pick, further cementing her reputation for combining rigorous science with compelling storytelling [1, 13].

Yet even as her young adult fiction career was flourishing, Dr. Kang was simultaneously developing a parallel track in adult historical fiction, and it is arguably in this genre that her unique combination of medical expertise and narrative craft has found its most perfect expression.

"A Beautiful Poison," published in 2017, marked Dr. Kang's debut in adult fiction and showcased her ability to weave together historical detail, medical accuracy, and murder mystery [4, 14]. Set in New York City during World War I and the Spanish flu pandemic of 1918, the novel follows three childhood friends—Allene, Jasper, and Birdie—who reunite as adults when a series of mysterious poisoning deaths threatens to destroy what remains of their fractured friendship. The novel drew directly on Dr. Kang's years at Bellevue Hospital and her research into the birth of forensic medicine in early twentieth-century New York [4].

Reviewers praised the book's sophisticated treatment of class and gender dynamics, with Elizabeth Blackwell, author of "In the Shadow of Lakecrest," describing it as: "An intriguing blend of history and suspense, A Beautiful Poison kept me guessing until the very end. Lydia Kang masterfully conjures up the world of early twentieth-century New York [1]." Jennifer Hillier, author of "Creep" and "The Butcher," called it "The perfect blend of mystery, history, and science" and "an entertaining read from beginning to end [1]." Dr. Kang had found a formula that worked beautifully: take a meticulously researched historical period, add characters navigating social constraints and personal trauma, introduce a medical or scientific mystery, and solve it with period-appropriate methods informed by genuine expertise.

She followed this success with "The Impossible Girl," in 2018, a historical thriller set in 1850s New York that explored the dark world of body snatching and early anatomical science [1, 15]. The novel's protagonist works secretly procuring bodies for medical students, navigating the moral ambiguities of a practice that, while gruesome, actually advanced medical knowledge at a time when legal cadaver procurement was nearly impossible.

"Opium and Absinthe," published in 2020, became one of Dr. Kang's most acclaimed works [1, 16]. Set in 1899 New York, the novel tells the story of Tillie Pembroke, a young woman from a wealthy family whose sister dies with mysterious bite wounds on her neck. As Tillie investigates, she becomes entangled in the world of substance use, addiction, and the supernatural, with Dracula's recent publication as a cultural backdrop. The novel allowed Dr. Kang to explore the history of substance misuse, the changing social acceptance of various drugs, and the scientific understanding of addiction; themes she would later expand upon in her nonfiction work and in speaking engagements about the stigma surrounding substance use disorder.

In 2022, Dr. Kang published "The Half-Life of Ruby Fielding," a historical mystery set during World War II that follows siblings Will and Maggie Scripps as they contribute to the war effort in Brooklyn [1, 17]. Will secretly scouts for the Manhattan Project while Maggie works at the Navy Yard, and both become embroiled in mysteries involving secret identities, wartime paranoia, and espionage.

Once again, Dr. Kang demonstrated her ability to ground fiction in meticulous historical and scientific research.

But perhaps Dr. Kang's most significant impact has come through her nonfiction work, co-authored with writer Nate Pedersen. In 2017, they published "Quackery: A Brief History of the Worst Ways to Cure Everything," a darkly humorous yet rigorously researched exploration of the medical "treatments" that humans have inflicted upon themselves through the ages [1, 18]. From leeches and mercury to lobotomies and radium water, the book catalogued the bizarre, dangerous, and sometimes well-intentioned but misguided therapies that once passed for medical care.

"Quackery, " was named a Science Friday Best Science Book of 2017 by NPR, introducing Dr. Kang to a broader audience of readers interested in medical history and scientific literacy [1, 19]. The book struck a perfect balance: entertaining enough to engage general readers, accurate enough to satisfy medical professionals, and thoughtful enough to raise important questions about how we distinguish legitimate medicine from pseudoscience, a question that remains urgently relevant in our age of medical misinformation.

The success of "Quackery" led to a second collaboration, "Patient Zero: A Curious History of the World's Worst Diseases," published in 2021 [1, 19, 20]. The timing could not have been more uncanny: Dr. Kang and Pedersen had begun researching and writing about pandemics in late 2019, before COVID-19 had entered public consciousness. In early January 2020, Dr. Kang mentioned in an email to her co-author that she'd seen articles about a SARS-like virus outbreak in Wuhan, China, wondering if it might make it into the book. She was doubtful that this particular outbreak would prove significant enough to merit inclusion.

Then Dr. Kang lived through what she was writing about. As an internal medicine physician in Omaha during the COVID-19 pandemic, she found herself simultaneously caring for COVID patients (including her own physician husband, who fell ill) and writing the chapter on the politicalization of pandemics [21]. "It was surreal," she later wrote. "But let's be honest; the entire pandemic has been surreal." She described the bizarre new normal of "COVID streaking," stripping off potentially contaminated clothes immediately upon arriving home, and the way the pandemic transformed everyday vocabulary with new verbs like "masking," "distancing," and "Zooming."

"Patient Zero" received a starred review from Publishers Weekly and won the 2022 Nebraska Book Award in the Nonfiction Popular History category [1, 22]. The book demonstrated Dr. Kang's ability to make complex medical and epidemiological concepts accessible to general readers while honoring the human stories behind disease outbreaks.

In 2025, Dr. Kang and Pedersen published their third nonfiction collaboration, "Pseudoscience: An Amusing History of Crackpot Ideas and Why We Love Them [23]." The book explores why humans are drawn to scientifically invalid ideas; from flat earth theory to the Ford Nucleon (a 1957 concept car that would have been powered by a small nuclear reactor) to rumpology (the practice of reading people's posteriors for fortune-telling purposes, reportedly coined by Sylvester Stallone's mother) [1, 23]. Rather than simply mocking pseudoscience, Dr. Kang and Pedersen take a more nuanced approach, examining why these ideas persist and what they reveal about human nature, our need for meaning, and our relationship with scientific authority.

Beyond these major works, Dr. Kang has contributed to numerous anthologies, demonstrating her versatility across genres and styles. Her short story appears in "Color Outside the Lines," a groundbreaking young adult anthology exploring interracial and LGBTQ+ relationships [1]. She contributed to the paranormal anthology that included stories exploring the darker aspects of human nature and supernatural horror. And notably, she became a Star Wars author, contributing the short story "Right-Hand Man" to the 2020 anthology "From a Certain Point of View: The Empire Strikes Back," which reimagines the iconic scene where the medical droid 2-1B attaches Luke Skywalker's prosthetic hand [1].

This entry into the Star Wars universe led to larger projects. In 2023, Dr. Kang published "Cataclysm, " a full-length novel set during the High Republic era of Star Wars, approximately 150 years before the events of "The Phantom Menace [1, 24]." The novel has been praised by Star Wars fans and critics alike, with StarWarsNews.net declaring that "Lydia Kang deserves all of the flowers, accolades, and recognition she can get because Cataclysm is as close to a Star Wars novel masterpiece as I can recall [25–27]." She has also contributed stories to other Star Wars anthologies, including "The Call of Coruscant" in "Star Wars: The High Republic Tales of Light and Life."

Her most recent young adult novel, "K-Jane," is scheduled for publication in late 2025 [1]. The book tells the story of a Korean American girl who doesn't feel "Korean enough" and decides to educate herself through K-pop, K-food, and K-drama, with predictably chaotic results. The novel represents Dr. Kang's continued exploration of identity, belonging, and the complex experience of navigating multiple cultural spaces.

Across approximately 12 published books spanning multiple genres—young adult science fiction, adult historical fiction, medical history, cultural commentary, and Star Wars novels—Dr. Kang has established herself as a uniquely versatile author whose medical expertise enriches everything she writes. But what truly distinguishes Dr. Kang in the literary world is her reputation for helping other writers achieve medical accuracy in their fiction. Recognizing that many authors struggle with medical scenarios, she began offering her expertise to fellow writers through her blog and social media, advising on everything from appropriate sedatives for specific situations to realistic timelines for recovery from injuries. She has been thanked in numerous acknowledgments sections and even appeared as a cameo character (Dr. Kang, naturally) in other authors' books [1, 7].

This generosity reflects a fundamental understanding that good fiction benefits from grounding in reality. Readers may accept dragons and faster-than-light travel, but they will be pulled out of a story if a character with a supposedly fatal wound is up and walking hours later, or if a medication produces effects inconsistent with its actual pharmacology. Dr. Kang's willingness to share her medical knowledge has helped elevate the quality of medical accuracy across contemporary fiction.

Her dual expertise has also made her a sought-after speaker. She has delivered talks on the history of medicine, the intersection of science and fiction, the importance of medical accuracy in storytelling, and the history of substance use and stigma [19]. At her alma mater, Roland Park Country School, where she delivered the 2025 Sarah Crane Cohen Visiting Scholar in the Humanities Lecture, she spoke to students about pursuing multiple passions, dealing with imposter syndrome, and the value of the scientific method in all aspects of life. "It was at Roland Park Country School that I learned I had a brain," she told the students, "and I had people around me who supported me for being smart."

Dr. Kang's impact on medicine extends beyond her clinical practice, though that work remains central to her identity. As an Associate Professor of Internal Medicine at the University of Nebraska Medical Center, she teaches and mentors medical students and residents. She has received multiple teaching awards, including the Top Teacher Award in 2014 and the Outstanding Dedication in Mentoring Award in 2017 from the Department of Internal Medicine [1, 2, 6, 19]. She has also contributed to medical literature through poetry and essays published in prestigious journals including JAMA, The Annals of Internal Medicine, the Canadian Medical Association Journal, and the Journal of General Internal Medicine. These pieces often explore the emotional and existential dimensions of medical practice; the experiences that don't fit neatly into progress notes or discharge summaries, but that constitute the actual texture of caring for sick and suffering people.

Her work in historical fiction serves an additional important function: it contextualizes contemporary medicine by revealing how we got here. When readers encounter the body snatchers of "The Impossible Girl," or the poisoners of "A Beautiful Poison, " or the substance users of "Opium and Absinthe," they gain perspective on how medical knowledge advances, often through ethically fraught means, and how social attitudes toward illness, death, and treatment evolve over time.

Similarly, her nonfiction books on quackery, pandemics, and pseudoscience serve as reminders that the boundary between legitimate medicine and harmful nonsense has always been contested, that scientific progress is hard-won and easily undermined, and that we ignore history at our peril. In our current era of vaccine hesitancy, medical misinformation on social media, and declining trust in scientific expertise, Dr. Kang's accessible, entertaining, yet scientifically rigorous books provide essential education disguised as entertainment.

Her characters often exist at the margins; genetically modified outcasts, body snatchers, addiction sufferers, people whose bodies or circumstances place them outside societal norms. This focus on the marginalized reflects both her medical practice (where she regularly encounters people failed by various systems) and her recognition that the most interesting stories often emerge from the spaces between categories, from people who don't fit neatly into prescribed boxes. As a Korean American woman in medicine and in publishing—two fields historically dominated by white men—Dr. Kang has navigated spaces where she might have felt pressure to downplay certain aspects of her identity. Yet her forthcoming novel "K-Jane," directly engages questions about cultural identity and belonging, suggesting her ongoing commitment to exploring these themes.

Dr. Kang currently balances her clinical practice, her teaching and mentoring responsibilities, her writing career spanning multiple genres, and her family life with her husband and three children (and two dogs, one of which she describes as looking "uncannily like an Ewok." How does she manage all of this? In presentations to students, she is remarkably honest about the difficulties. She speaks about imposter syndrome, about the challenge of balancing dual careers and family, about pursuing passions despite setbacks and fear. Her message to aspiring physician-writers and to young people trying to navigate multiple interests is not that it's easy, but that it's possible, and that the integration of different passions can create something more interesting than choosing just one path.

This honesty is one of Dr. Kang's greatest gift to her readers and to the medical community. She does not present herself as having achieved some perfect work-life balance or as possessing some special talent that makes her dual career easy. Instead, she shows up as someone who loves both medicine and writing, who refuses to give up either, and who does the hard work of making both possible, while understanding that "possible" doesn't mean "effortless."

References

1. Kang L. Lydia Kang [Official website]. n.d. https://lydiakang.com/.
2. University of Nebraska Medical Center. Lydia Kang, MD. Department of Internal Medicine Faculty Profile. n.d. https://www.unmc.edu/intmed/divisions/gim/faculty/kang.html.
3. Penguin Random House. Lydia Kang [Author page]. n.d. https://www.penguinrandomhouse.com/authors/239558/lydia-kang/.
4. Finck M. Q&A with Lydia Kang. Women Writers, Women's Books; 2017, October 5. https://booksbywomen.org/qa-with-lydia-kang-by-mm-finck/.
5. Doximity. Dr. Lydia Kang, MD. n.d. https://www.doximity.com/pub/lydia-kang-md.
6. McGoogan Library News. Miracle to menace: a conversation with Dr. Lydia Kang. 2024, October 24 https://blog.unmc.edu/library/2024/10/24/miracle-to-menace-a-conversation-with-dr-lydia-kang/.
7. Omaha Magazine. Lydia Kang is in Control. 2013, December 16. https://www.omahamagazine.com/lifestyle/lydia-kang-is-in-control/.
8. University of Nebraska Medical Center Newsroom. UNMC's Lydia Kang, M.D., to read from her novels. 2016, February 23. https://www.unmc.edu/newsroom/2016/02/23/unmcs-lydia-kang-m-d-to-read-from-her-novels/.
9. University of Nebraska Medical Center Newsroom. Dr. Kang to hold reading from her book, 'Patient Zero.' 2022, April 15. https://www.unmc.edu/newsroom/2022/04/15/dr-kang-to-hold-reading-from-her-book-patient-zero/.
10. Kang L. Control. New York: Dial Books; 2013.
11. Kang L. Catalyst. New York: Dial Books; 2015.
12. Kang L. The November girl. New York: Entangled Publishing; 2017.
13. Kang L. Toxic. New York: Entangled Publishing; 2018.
14. Kang L. A beautiful poison. Seattle: Lake Union Publishing; 2017.
15. Kang L. The impossible girl. Seattle: Lake Union Publishing; 2018.
16. Kang L. Opium and absinthe. Seattle: Lake Union Publishing; 2020.

17. Kang L. The half-life of ruby fielding. Seattle: Lake Union Publishing; 2022.
18. Kang L, Pedersen N. Quackery: a brief history of the worst ways to cure everything. New York: Workman Publishing; 2017.
19. Hachette Speakers Bureau. Dr. Lydia Kang. n.d. https://hachettespeakersbureau.com/dr-lydia-kang/.
20. Kang L, Pedersen N. Patient zero: a curious history of the world's worst diseases. New York: Workman Publishing; 2021.
21. Flatwater Free Press. A Nebraska doctor was writing a history of nightmare pandemics. Then she lived one. 2021, October 29. https://flatwaterfreepress.org/a-nebraska-doctor-was-writing-a-history-of-nightmare-pandemics-then-she-lived-one/.
22. Nebraska Center for the Book. Nebraska Book Award winners. n.d. https://centerforthebook.nebraska.gov/awards/winners/nebook.html.
23. Kang L, Pedersen N. Pseudoscience: an amusing history of crackpot ideas and why we love them. New York: Workman/Hachette; 2025.
24. Kang L. Cataclysm (Star Wars: The High Republic). New York: Random House Worlds; 2023.
25. University of Nebraska Medical Center Newsroom. Never tell her the odds. 2022, November 29. https://www.unmc.edu/newsroom/2022/11/29/never-tell-her-the-odds/.
26. Star Wars News Net. Review: Lydia Kang delivers a High Republic masterpiece in 'Star Wars: Cataclysm.' 2023, April 3. https://www.starwarsnewsnet.com/2023/04/review-lydia-kang-delivers-a-high-republic-masterpiece-in-star-wars-cataclysm.html.
27. Dork Side of the Force. Review: Star Wars: The High Republic: Cataclysm by Lydia Kang. 2023, April 4. https://dorksideoftheforce.com/2023/04/04/review-lydia-kangs-cataclysm-incredibly-intense-convergence-violence-high-republic-jedi/.

Chapter 14
Tess Gerritsen, MD

In the Fall of 21, every Monday at 10 o'clock, a group of friends and I would gather in my college apartment with beverages and snacks to watch two women solve Boston's toughest crimes. Detective Jane Rizzoli and Dr. Maura Isles were witty protagonists who took on, sometimes gruesome, challenges to serve crisp justice on cable television. And while crime dramas were certainly not new, in a world of Law and Order, Rizzoli & Isles challenged the heteronormative standard while focusing on the gritty mechanics of the justice system and the medical examiner's office. The show's end coincided with my second year of medical school, when a medical examiner was invited to discuss his work, as well as the field of Forensic Pathology, with my class. He began by asking us what we knew about the medical examiner's office. An enterprising student volunteered "SVU," while I, close to the front, muttered "Rizzoli and Isles." "Written by a doctor, did you know?" he returned with a grin.

I hadn't known. To be accurate, Dr. Tess Gerritsen's 13 book series of the eponymous characters inspired the television show on TNT [1]. Her dark mystery series was a creation meant to depict the vicissitudes of the professional woman, who rolls up her sleeves for exacting work, and she even hinted that the creation of Dr. Isles was something of a self-portrait [1]. I would dive into her work, adding first *The Surgeon*, and then *The Apprentice* to my Kindle, saving the latter for my post-USMLE break before my third year. I will admit to being smitten with Dr. Gerritsen's style; she has the perfect stark artistry that is necessary for thrillers and the surgical calm intrinsic to good suspense. It is my pleasure to share her work with you.

Dr. Tess Gerritsen was born Terry Tom on June 12, 1953, in San Diego, California, the daughter of a Chinese immigrant mother and a Chinese-American father who worked as a seafood chef [2, 3]. Growing up in a first-generation immigrant household, she experienced the particular pressures familiar to many children of immigrants: high expectations for academic achievement, parental skepticism about impractical career paths, and the weight of proving oneself in a culture that didn't always make space for people who looked like her [1–3].

O. M. Cox, *The Pen, The Stethoscope, and The Scalpel*,
https://doi.org/10.1007/978-3-032-19406-0_14

As a child, young Terry devoured Nancy Drew mysteries, dreaming of one day writing her own detective novels [2, 4]. She would lose herself in these stories, captivated by the clever teenage sleuth who solved crimes through intelligence and persistence. But when she expressed her desire to become a writer, her family's response was predictable: writing was not a stable career, not a path to security [1, 2]. Her family encouraged her toward medicine instead; a respectable profession, a guaranteed income, a way to honor the sacrifices they had made [2].

So, Terry Tom, the girl who dreamed of writing mysteries, became a pre-med student. But her intellectual curiosity ranged wider than biology and chemistry. At Stanford University, she chose to major in anthropology, fascinated by the ranges of human behavior, the patterns of culture, the mysteries of why people do what they do [1, 5]. She graduated Phi Beta Kappa in 1975 with her B.A. in Anthropology, having spent time cataloguing centuries-old human remains, an early exposure to death and the stories bodies tell that would later inform her fiction [2].

From Stanford, she proceeded to the University of California, San Francisco, for medical school, earning her M.D. in 1979 [1, 2, 6]. She completed her internal medicine residency and began practicing as a physician in Honolulu, Hawaii. For nearly a decade, she lived the life her family had envisioned for her: Dr. Terry Tom, internist, a successful Chinese-American woman who had achieved the American dream through education and hard work.

In 1977, during medical school, she married Jacob Gerritsen, who was also a physician [2]. Together they would build a medical household, eventually having two sons, Joshua and Adam [1, 4]. It seemed Terry had settled into the predictable trajectory of a physician's life: practice medicine, raise children, perhaps eventually join her husband in a comfortable private practice or academic position.

But the dream of writing had never died. While on maternity leave after the birth of one of her sons, Dr. Gerritsen found herself with a rare commodity: time to think, time to imagine, time to finally try her hand at the fiction she had always wanted to write. She began writing, at first tentatively, then with growing confidence and commitment [1, 2, 4, 6].

On a whim, she submitted a literary short story to *Honolulu Magazine's* statewide fiction contest. To her amazement and delight, she won first place [2, 4]. The validation was intoxicating proof that she had talent; that her secret dream might not be foolish after all. Encouraged by this success, she decided to try her hand at a full-length novel. Her first two novels went unpublished; what she would later call her "practice novels," essential work that honed her craft [2, 4]. But in 1986, she sold "Call After Midnight," a romantic thriller, to Harlequin Intrigue. The book was published in 1987, launching her professional writing career [1, 2, 6].

There was a practical consideration in her choice of genre: Dr. Gerritsen had enjoyed reading romance novels during her years in medical practice, finding them an escape from the stress of patient care. Writing in the romance genre also made commercial sense; Harlequin published prolifically and paid advances. And there was the matter of her byline. Her given name, Terry, was gender-ambiguous, and in the romance genre, readers expected female authors. And so, Terry Tom Gerritsen feminized her first name to Tess, the pen name she would use for the rest of her career [2, 4].

For the next 9 years, Dr. Gerritsen published romantic suspense novels through Harlequin Intrigue and Harper Paperbacks. Titles like "Never Say Die (1992)," "Keeper of the Bride" (1996), and others gained her a solid following in the romance community [2, 4]. She won Romantic Times Reviewers' Choice awards for best Harlequin Intrigue novel. She even co-wrote the screenplay for "Adrift," which aired as a CBS Movie of the Week in 1993, starring Kate Jackson and Bruce Greenwood [1, 2, 6]. But Dr. Gerritsen was growing restless with the romance genre. Her medical background, her intellectual curiosity, her fascination with the darker aspects of human nature; all of these pulled her toward a different kind of storytelling. She wanted to write something more serious, something that drew on her professional expertise, something that would allow her to explore the moral complexities and visceral realities of medicine.

The catalyst came, as so many story ideas do, from a chance encounter. At a dinner party, Dr. Gerritsen found herself seated next to an ex-cop who ran a security service protecting American businessmen in Russia. He told her a horrifying story: young orphans were vanishing from the streets of Moscow, and police believed the children were being kidnapped and shipped abroad as organ donors for wealthy patients willing to pay exorbitant sums and ask no questions [2, 5].

The story haunted Dr. Gerritsen. She immediately called her brother-in-law, a reporter for *Newsweek*, urging him to investigate. *Newsweek* was unable to track down proof of the organ trafficking ring, but Dr. Gerritsen couldn't stop thinking about those missing Russian orphans, couldn't shake the horror of children being harvested for their organs. She began researching the black market in human organs, the desperate patients who turned to illegal sources, and the ethical nightmares of transplant medicine [1].

Those missing children became the inspiration for "Harvest, " published in 1996 [2, 5]. The novel marked a dramatic departure from her earlier work; this was a medical thriller, dark and violent, exploring the murky intersection of medicine, crime, and desperation. The plot follows Dr. Abby DiMatteo, a surgical resident at a Boston hospital, who stumbles upon a sinister organ transplant conspiracy and must fight to expose it while staying alive.

"Harvest," was Dr. Gerritsen's first hardcover novel, a step up in prestige from her previous mass-market paperbacks [1, 2, 6]. More significantly, it debuted at number 13 on the *New York Times* bestseller list [1]. Success validated her instinct that her medical knowledge combined with her storytelling ability could produce something commercially successful and artistically satisfying. Film rights sold to Paramount/Dreamworks, and the book was translated into 20 foreign languages.

Publishers Weekly dubbed her the "medical suspense queen," a title that acknowledged her unique position: a physician who could write about medical settings with authority and insider knowledge, who knew what an autopsy room smelled like, what it felt like to hold a scalpel, what doctors actually said to each other when patients weren't present [7].

Dr. Gerritsen followed "Harvest" with more medical thrillers: "Life Support" (1997), which explored the ethics of anti-aging treatments and the fear of prion diseases like Mad Cow Disease; "Bloodstream" (1998); and "Gravity" (1999), a thriller set on the International Space Station that demonstrated her range beyond hospital settings [1, 4]. Each book built her reputation as a writer who could combine medical accuracy with pulse-pounding suspense. She studied scientific journals and magazines to research her novels, aiming to be, in her words, "a futurist," who anticipated medical developments. "It's what's happening in the labs right now that will be practiced twenty years from now," she explained. "I want my books to look ahead."

But her most enduring contribution to popular culture would come with her next major shift, from medical thrillers to crime procedurals. In 2001, Dr. Gerritsen published "The Surgeon," a novel about a serial killer who stalks women in their homes, attacking them with surgical precision [1, 2, 8]. The book introduced Boston homicide detective Jane Rizzoli, though curiously, Rizzoli was only a secondary character in this first book, overshadowed by Dr. Catherine Cordell, a trauma surgeon who had survived an attack by a similar killer 2 years earlier.

Readers and Dr. Gerritsen herself were drawn to Jane Rizzoli. Here was a character unlike the typical romance heroine or even the typical female detective: tough, working-class, Italian-American, sarcastic, brilliant but insecure, fighting for respect in a male-dominated profession. Rizzoli was short, dark-haired, and explicitly described as not conventionally beautiful; a radical choice in a literary landscape that typically made female protagonists attractive even when portraying them as tough.

"The Surgeon," won the RITA Award for Best Romantic Suspense Novel in 2002, despite having moved far from traditional romance [1, 2, 9]. Dr. Gerritsen was transitioning into a new genre, and this award recognized that readers were following her there.

The sequel, "The Apprentice," (2002), brought back both the imprisoned killer Warren Hoyt and Detective Rizzoli, now promoted to the Homicide unit [1, 2, 10]. More significantly, it introduced Dr. Maura Isles, Boston's chief medical examiner [2]. Dr. Isles was everything Rizzoli was not: tall, elegant, cool, controlled, supremely competent, unfailingly polite. Where Rizzoli was emotional and intuitive, Isles was analytical and detached. Where Rizzoli came from working-class Italian roots, Isles was raised in an upper-middle-class household [10].

Dr. Gerritsen has admitted that Isles, like her creator, is a physician who brought precision and scientific rigor to her work. Like Isles, Dr. Gerritsen is comfortable in the world of death and pathology, able to look at gruesome crime scenes with clinical detachment. And like Isles, she exists somewhat outside the mainstream, her scientific knowledge and immigrant background setting her apart.

The pairing of Rizzoli and Isles proved irresistible. Over the next 20 years, Dr. Gerritsen would publish 13 novels in the series (as of 2022's "Listen to Me") [1, 2]. Each book featured the two women investigating cases that ranged from serial killers to international conspiracies, from ancient Chinese martial arts secrets to disappearances in the Wyoming wilderness.

The series titles tell their own story: "The Sinner" (2003), "Body Double" (2004), "Vanish" (2005), "The Mephisto Club" (2006), "The Keepsake" (2008), "Ice Cold" (2010), "The Silent Girl" (2011), "Last to Die" (2012), "Die Again" (2014), and "I Know a Secret" (2017) [1, 2, 8, 10–12]. Each explored different facets of medical and criminal investigation, each deepened the relationship between the two protagonists, each demonstrated Dr. Gerritsen's command of suspense and pacing.

"Vanish" won the Nero Wolfe Award for Best Mystery Novel in 2006 and was nominated for both an Edgar Award and a Macavity Award [1, 2, 11]. Critics compared Dr. Gerritsen favorably to other titans of medical suspense. Stephen King said she was "even better than Michael Crichton [1]." James Patterson praised her work. The Chicago Tribune called her prose "polished and riveting [1]." The Philadelphia Inquirer deemed her books "pulse-pounding fun [1]."

In 2009, TNT picked up the rights to adapt the Rizzoli & Isles series for television. The show premiered in July 2010, starring Angie Harmon as Detective Jane Rizzoli and Sasha Alexander as Dr. Maura Isles [13]. The series ran for seven seasons, from 2010 to 2016, becoming one of TNT's most-watched programs and introducing Dr. Gerritsen's characters to millions of viewers who might never have picked up one of her books [13–15].

The television adaptation took liberties with the source material; the show emphasized the friendship between the two women, softened some of the darker edges of the novels, and diverged significantly from book plots after the first season. Dr. Gerritsen made a cameo appearance in the series' final season as a writer helping Maura Isles establish herself in the literary world, a meta moment that acknowledged the series' origins [2].

The impact of the television show on Dr. Gerritsen's book sales was dramatic. The series brought her work to international audiences, particularly in Europe and Asia, where she became a major bestseller. She found herself mobbed by fans at book signings, needing security details at events. When she attended the Istanbul Book Fair, hundreds of fans lined up to meet her. "Now I sort of understand what 'it's like to be a rock star,'"she said. "It was sort of overwhelming [16]."

Throughout the Rizzoli & Isles series, Dr. Gerritsen continued to demonstrate the value of her medical training. Her descriptions of autopsy procedures are clinically accurate; the Y-incision, the removal of organs, the weight and appearance of diseased tissue, the smells and sounds of the morgue. Readers who work in medicine appreciate these details; readers without medical background find them simultaneously horrifying and fascinating.

More importantly, her medical knowledge allows her to construct plausible murder mysteries. The methods of killing, the forensic evidence, the medical examiner's deductions; all ring true because Dr. Gerritsen understands the science. She knows how long it takes for rigor mortis to set in, what different types of wounds look like, how toxicology screens work, which poisons are detectable, and which aren't.

But Dr. Gerritsen is careful not to let medical detail overwhelm narrative. She has said she writes for someone who wants the story to move, who doesn't need three pages of atmospheric description when a few well-chosen details will do. Even as she built the Rizzoli & Isles empire, Dr. Gerritsen occasionally stepped outside the series to write standalone novels. “The Bone Garden,” (2007) is a historical thriller set in 1830s Boston, exploring the grisly world of medical grave robbers and featuring a character based on Dr. Oliver Wendell Holmes [1, 2]. The book allowed her to combine her love of history, her medical knowledge, and her thriller-writing skills in a gothic tale of murder and medicine.

“Playing with Fire” (2015) is a supernatural thriller about a violinist who discovers a haunting piece of music—the Incendio waltz—in a Roman antiques shop [1, 17]. Dr. Gerritsen, who plays the violin herself, actually composed the Incendio waltz for the novel; it has been performed and recorded by professional violinists, a remarkable example of multimedia artistic creation [1, 18–20]. “The Shape of Night” (2019) is a paranormal gothic romance about a woman fleeing to coastal Maine who finds herself involved with both a serial killer investigation and the ghost of a sea captain. The novel allowed Dr. Gerritsen to return to her romance roots while incorporating the suspense elements she had mastered in her thrillers [1, 6].

Most recently, Dr. Gerritsen has launched a new series. “The Spy Coast” (2023) introduces Maggie Bird, a retired CIA operative trying to live quietly in a small Maine coastal town until enemies from her past threaten everything she’s built [1]. The novel was inspired by Dr. Gerritsen’s own life in Camden, Maine, where she discovered that several of her neighbors were retired intelligence operatives [1, 21]. “I’d see gray-haired people in the grocery store and post office, and I wondered about their past exploits,” she explained. “Surely they had stories to tell! [9]” The book introduces the Martini Club, a group of retired spies who meet under the cover of being a book club [12]. Amazon Studios has acquired the rights to develop the novel for television, potentially launching another franchise for Dr. Gerritsen. A sequel, “The Summer Guests” (2024), continues Maggie Bird’s adventures [1, 5].

Dr. Gerritsen has also ventured into filmmaking. In 2018, she and her son Josh produced “Island Zero,” a horror movie. In 2022, they created “Magnificent Beast,” a documentary exploring the origins of religious dietary restrictions around pork [1]. These projects demonstrate her continued creative restlessness, her refusal to be limited to a single medium.

Over her 37-year writing career, Dr. Gerritsen has published over 30 novels [1]. Her books have sold over 40 million copies worldwide and been translated into more than 40 languages [6]. She has won multiple awards including the RITA, the Nero Wolfe Award, and numerous Romantic Times Reviewers’ Choice Awards [1].

The question of her impact on medicine is complex. Unlike some physician-authors who continue clinical practice while writing, Dr. Gerritsen retired from medicine to write full-time [1, 4]. She left patient care behind to pursue her creative work, a decision that might seem like abandoning one career for another. But I would argue that her impact on medicine comes through a different channel: she has shaped how millions of people understand medical examiners, forensic pathology, and the scientific investigation of death. Through Maura Isles, she has made the work of medical examiners visible and comprehensible to a general audience. She has shown that forensic pathology requires not just strong stomachs but brilliant analytical minds, that medical examiners are physicians who continue to serve the dead and seek justice for them.

The Rizzoli & Isles television series, in particular, has influenced how people perceive forensic pathology and may have inspired some viewers to pursue careers in the field; much as the CSI franchise did for crime scene investigation. Dr. Gerritsen has brought respect and glamour to a medical specialty that is often overlooked, that struggles to recruit despite its importance to the justice system. Moreover, her meticulous research and medical accuracy have raised the bar for medical thrillers generally. Other authors know they're competing with a former physician who gets the details right. This has pushed the entire genre toward greater authenticity, which benefits readers and creates more realistic portrayals of medical professionals in popular culture.

She has also contributed essays to volumes published by Mystery Writers of America and International Thriller Writers, sharing her expertise about constructing medical mysteries [4]. She blogs regularly about the writing business, offering advice to aspiring authors. In this way, she continues to teach, much as she might have taught medical students if she had pursued an academic medicine career.

Her protagonists are almost always women; women doctors, women detectives, women who are competent professionals navigating male-dominated fields while also dealing with personal struggles, relationship challenges, and societal expectations. In the 1990s and 2000s, this representation mattered, is it continues to do today. Dr. Gerritsen showed that women could be brilliant surgeons and tough detectives, that they could be the heroes rather than solely the victims or love interests.

The Rizzoli & Isles series, in particular, has had significant cultural impact. The relationship between the two women—professional partnership, deep friendship, and something that many fans read as having romantic undertones—challenged heteronormative assumptions about female relationships on television. While the show never made the relationship explicitly romantic, it also never gave either woman a sustained, satisfying heterosexual romance. The emotional center of the series was always the bond between the two women.

Dr. Gerritsen's Chinese-American heritage has also informed her work. "The Silent Girl," (2011) explores Boston's Chinatown and incorporates Chinese martial arts and cultural elements [1]. The novel features a Chinese chef as one of the victims and delves into Chinese mythology and philosophy. This book draws directly on stories Dr. Gerritsen's mother told her as a child—traditional Chinese tales about the Monkey King and other figures from Chinese folklore.

In interviews, Dr. Gerritsen has spoken about the challenge of being a Chinese-American woman in publishing, about assumptions people make when they see her name or her face before reading her work, about the pressure to write "Asian stories" or alternatively to avoid "ethnic content" to appeal to mainstream audiences [1]. She has navigated these pressures with grace, writing primarily mainstream thrillers while occasionally incorporating her heritage when it serves the story.

Now in her 70s, Dr. Gerritsen lives in Camden, Maine, a picturesque coastal town that has become the setting for some of her recent work. She enjoys gardening and playing the fiddle; pursuits that offer respite from the dark imaginings required to create convincing serial killers and murder mysteries. She remains married to Jacob, her physician husband of nearly 50 years [1, 21].

For aspiring physician-writers, for readers who love intelligent thrillers, for anyone who has ever been told their dream was impractical and pursued it anyway; Dr. Tess Gerritsen's career stands as inspiration and proof that it is possible to live multiple lives, to honor multiple callings, to bring your whole self to your work.

References

1. Gerritsen T. About. Tess Gerritsen Official Website. n.d. https://www.tessgerritsen.com/about.
2. EBSCO Research Starters. Tess Gerritsen. n.d. https://www.ebsco.com/research-starters/biography/tess-gerritsen.
3. Harnett L. Author Tess Gerritsen's life takes an unexpected turn. Portsmouth Herald. 2005, September 18. https://www.seacoastonline.com/story/entertainment/local/2005/09/18/author-tess-gerritsen-s-life/50235767007/.
4. Goodreads. Tess Gerritsen (Author of The Surgeon). n.d. https://www.goodreads.com/author/show/18149.Tess_Gerritsen.
5. Fantastic Fiction. Tess Gerritsen. n.d. https://www.fantasticfiction.com/g/tess-gerritsen/.
6. Amazon. Tess Gerritsen: books, biography. n.d. https://www.amazon.com/stores/Tess%20Gerritsen/author/B000AQ4IHU.
7. Publishers Weekly. All danger and glamour: PW talks with Tess Gerritsen. 2024, October 14. https://www.publishersweekly.com/pw/by-topic/authors/interviews/article/96146-all-danger-and-glamour-pw-talks-with-tess-gerritsen.html.
8. Gerritsen T. The surgeon. Ballantine Books; New York, NY. 2001.
9. LibraryThing. Author interview: Tess Gerritsen. 2025, March. https://blog.librarything.com/2025/03/author-interview-tess-gerritsen/.
10. Gerritsen T. The apprentice. Ballantine Books; New York, NY. 2002.
11. Gerritsen T. Vanish. Ballantine Books; New York, NY. 2005.
12. Gerritsen T. The spy coast. Thomas & Mercer; Seattle, WA. 2023.
13. IMDb. Rizzoli & Isles (TV series 2010–2016). n.d. https://www.imdb.com/title/tt1551632.
14. Deadline. 'Rizzoli & Isles' to end after seven seasons. 2016, January 7. https://deadline.com/2016/01/rizzoli-isles-canceled-7-seasons-1201677729/.
15. Screen Rant. NCIS star Sasha Alexander's underrated crime drama Rizzoli & Isles resurges on streaming. 2025, August. https://screenrant.com/ncis-sasha-alexander-rizzoli-isles-peacock-streaming-charts-success/.
16. Silverman J. Tess Gerritsen author interview. BookBrowse; 2015. https://www.bookbrowse.com/author_interviews/full/index.cfm/author_number/805/tess-gerritsen#interview.
17. Gerritsen T. Playing with fire. Ballantine Books; New York, NY. 2015.
18. Waterstones. 'Incendio': the story behind the music by Tess Gerritsen. n.d. https://www.waterstones.com/blog/incendio-the-story-behind-the-music-by-tess-gerritsen.
19. The Big Thrill. Playing with fire: Between the lines with Tess Gerritsen. 2015, November. https://www.thebigthrill.org/2015/11/between-the-lines-with-tess-gerritsen-on-playing-with-fire-interview-by-dawn-ius/.
20. Boston Globe. Maine author Tess Gerritsen wrote a thriller and a creepy song to go with it.2015, November 15. https://www.bostonglobe.com/arts/books/2015/11/15/maine-author-tess-gerritsen-wrote-thriller-and-creepy-song-with/.
21. BookTrib. Tess Gerritsen interview: The Spy Coast. 2023, November 8. https://booktrib.com/2023/11/08/tess-gerritsen-interview-the-spy-coast/.

Chapter 15
Lori Arviso Alvord, MD

Woven into the core curriculum of our pre-clinical years of medical education was a class titled "Practice of Medicine," affectionally known as "POM." In POM sessions we learned and performed physical exams, interviewed standardized patients who were community members with a skill for acting, and began to document our findings in the style of a physician in training. We also broke apart into small groups where clinical cases were reviewed for analysis of technique, differential and outcomes. It was also during these small group sessions that we collectively examined our role and responsibility as future physicians when faced with patient cultural practices. The words "cultural competence," were being phased out for a more realistic "cultural awareness," and we were exposed to a variety of cases requiring navigation of a family's customs, whether religious, geographic or cultural. The expectation following graduation was not that we would become experts of the innumerable patient practices we might encounter, but that we would be more understanding of the potential impact these traditions have on patient adherence with recommendations, tolerance of medication and agreement with treatment plans. There is evidence to suggest that this practice makes us all better listeners, better patient advocates, and better doctors. And while it is impossible to encounter and learn from all potential patient cultures, there are physicians among us who have the valuable insight provided by lived experience. They are more easily able to connect the patient perspective with the evidence-based treatment regimen, and simultaneously anticipate queries borne from lived identity. In Dr. Lori Alvord's literary work, there is the unique opportunity to imbibe of such cultural lessons focusing on the Native American Dine'é tribe. I am excited to share her work here.

Dr. Lori Arviso Alvord was born in 1958 in Crownpoint, New Mexico, a small town on the Navajo reservation, located approximately 130 miles from Albuquerque in one of the more remote corners of the American Southwest [1–3]. She is a member of the Tsinnaajinii' clan (also known as the Black Streaked Wood or Ponderosa Pine clan) through her father and the Ashihii' Diné (Salt People) clan through her mother [1, 2]. In Navajo tradition, clan membership is everything; it determines

O. M. Cox, *The Pen, The Stethoscope, and The Scalpel*,
https://doi.org/10.1007/978-3-032-19406-0_15

relationships, responsibilities, and one's place in the intricate web of kinship that holds the Diné people together. Young Lori would introduce herself this way, paying homage to her maternal and paternal lineage, as is customary among tribal members [1].

Her father, Robert Cupp, was Diné; her mother, Rita Colgan, was White [4]. This bicultural heritage meant that Lori grew up navigating two very different worlds from the beginning. English was the first language spoken in her home, which was unusual for Navajo families of that era but would later prove advantageous in her academic pursuits [1, 3]. Yet despite the linguistic assimilation, her family remained deeply connected to Navajo culture and traditions. Her shinaalii (maternal grandmother) taught her about the Navajo way of life, the ancient stories, and the concept of hózhó (pronounced ho-ZHO); the Navajo philosophy of living in balance, harmony, and beauty [1].

Growing up on the reservation in the 1960s and 1970s, Lori saw little that suggested a future in medicine. She had no exposure to Navajo physicians or other professionals; they simply didn't exist in her immediate world [1]. Her parents, though loving and supportive, did not have college degrees themselves. The path from a remote reservation town to the halls of an elite medical school seemed not just difficult but nearly impossible to imagine. And yet, something in the younger Lori yearned for more, even if she couldn't quite articulate what that more might be.

She graduated from Crownpoint High School and, through hard work and determination, was accepted to Dartmouth College in Hanover, New Hampshire [1, 4, 5]. The culture shock was profound. Dartmouth, an Ivy League institution founded in 1769, could not have been more different from the Navajo reservation. While Dartmouth had been established partially to educate Native Americans, by the time Lori arrived in the late 1970s, Native students were a tiny minority navigating an overwhelmingly white, privileged environment [1, 4].

Lori initially majored in natural sciences, drawn by a fascination with how things worked, how bodies functioned, how the natural world operated according to discoverable principles. But she struggled with the science courses, receiving low grades that shook her confidence [3–5]. In Navajo culture, direct eye contact is often avoided out of respect, and touching strangers—particularly across gender lines—is considered inappropriate. These cultural norms conflicted sharply with the expectations of medical education, where students must look patients in the eye, touch bodies, and develop an easy familiarity with physical examination [4].

After receiving several disappointing grades, Lori concluded that she simply wasn't smart enough for a STEM career. The imposter syndrome that plagues so many first-generation college students, particularly those from minoritized communities, convinced her that science was not her path. She switched to a double major in psychology and sociology, modified with a focus on Native American studies; fields that allowed her to explore human behavior and cultural patterns from a less technically demanding angle [2, 3, 5]. She graduated from Dartmouth cum laude in 1979, having found intellectual satisfaction even if not in the field she had initially imagined [2, 5].

After graduation, needing work and uncertain about her next steps, Lori took a position as a research assistant at the Veterans Administration clinic in Albuquerque, New Mexico [3–5]. It was there, working on a neurobiology research team, that her life changed direction. A neuroanatomy course had sparked something in her during college: a deep interest in neurology that she hadn't fully recognized at the time. Now, surrounded by physicians and researchers, she found herself increasingly drawn to medical questions. The doctors she worked with saw something in her, a sharp analytical mind and a genuine curiosity about disease and healing.

One of the doctors coordinating research in the lab pulled her aside one day and suggested she should consider medical school [3, 5]. Lori hesitated at the suggestion. Medical school? After her struggles with science at Dartmouth? It seemed absurd. But the doctor was insistent; she had what it took, he said. She just needed to believe in herself.

Tentatively, Lori enrolled at the University of New Mexico to retake pre-med courses. This time, perhaps because she was older, more mature, or simply more determined, she excelled [4, 5]. The difference was remarkable; the same subjects that had defeated her at Dartmouth now made sense. She applied to medical schools and was accepted to Stanford University School of Medicine, one of the most prestigious medical programs in the country [1, 3, 5].

Stanford, like Dartmouth before it, represented a dramatic cultural transition. In 1981, when Lori began medical school, women comprised only about 25% of medical students nationwide, and Native American students were vanishingly rare. The surgical world she would eventually enter was even more homogeneous; in the early 1980s, only 6% of surgeons were women, and only a handful were Native American [6].

At Stanford, Lori met Dr. Ron Lujan, a Native American general surgeon from the Taos and San Juan Pueblo Tribes. Dr. Lujan became a mentor and guide, teaching her about surgical procedures and patient care before her formal surgical rotations even began [1, 7]. His presence—proof that a Native American could succeed in surgery—was invaluable. He showed her the ropes, helped her navigate the unspoken cultural codes of academic medicine, and demonstrated surgical techniques with patience and care.

Medical School posed specific challenges for Lori beyond the academic rigor. Navajo tradition holds that touching dead bodies brings disharmony and danger, yet gross anatomy, with its required dissection of cadavers, is a cornerstone of medical education [3, 8]. Navajo healers avoid cutting into the body when possible; surgery violates fundamental principles about the sanctity and wholeness of the human form. Each time Lori entered the anatomy lab or the operating room, she was transgressing boundaries that her culture had established for good reasons, rooted in centuries of wisdom about health, harmony, and the interconnectedness of all things.

But Lori persisted. When she completed her core surgery clerkship, she impressed her attending physicians so thoroughly that she received honors and was invited to apply to Stanford's general surgery residency program; a highly competitive position that typically went to the top candidates from the nation's best medical schools.

She was accepted and embarked on a grueling six-year surgical residency at Stanford University Hospital, serving as Chief Resident from 1990 to 1991 [5, 9, 10].

In 1994, Dr. Lori Arviso Alvord earned her board certification in general surgery, becoming the first Navajo woman—indeed, the first Diné woman—ever to achieve this distinction [1, 3, 9, 11]. It was a historic accomplishment, the culmination of years of struggle against cultural barriers, gender discrimination, and her own self-doubt. One might think this would be the triumphant conclusion of her story: reservation girl overcomes all odds, becomes surgeon, achieves the American dream. But for Dr. Alvord, board certification was not an ending but a beginning; the start of a more complex and ultimately more meaningful journey.

From 1991 to 1997, Dr. Alvord practiced as a surgeon with the Indian Health Service at the Gallup Indian Medical Center in New Mexico, returning to serve the very community she had grown up in [1–3, 5]. She had left the reservation as a girl with uncertain prospects; she returned as a highly trained surgeon with the skills to save lives. It should have been a simple homecoming.

But Dr. Alvord quickly realized that her technical surgical skills, impressive as they were, were not sufficient to truly heal her patients [1]. The Navajo people she cared for were often frightened of her Western approach; the sometimes cold, always efficient manner she had cultivated at Stanford, the emphasis on quick diagnosis and rapid intervention, and the focus on the diseased organ rather than the whole person. They brought with them beliefs about illness that had nothing to do with bacteria or tumors and everything to do with harmony, balance, relationships, and spiritual wellness [1].

One patient might express concerns that his gallbladder problems stemmed from violating a taboo or from disharmony in his family relationships. Another might want to undergo a traditional healing ceremony before or after surgery. Still others might refuse certain procedures or medications because they conflicted with Navajo teachings. Dr. Alvord, trained in the reductionist, mechanistic model of Western medicine, initially struggled to take these beliefs seriously [1]. She had learned to see the body as a machine that could be repaired; replace this part, remove that blockage, cut out the diseased tissue. But her patients saw their bodies as inseparable from their minds, spirits, relationships, and environment.

It was humbling and deeply challenging. Dr. Alvord, who had worked so hard to master Western surgical techniques, now had to learn a completely different approach to healing; one that her own culture had been practicing for centuries but which she had never formally studied. She went back to the traditional healers of her tribe, the hataali (medicine men), to learn what a surgical residency could not teach her [1].

From the Navajo healers, Dr. Alvord heard a resounding message: everything in life is connected. Illness and healing alike come from maintaining strong and healthy relationships in every aspect of our lives, with family, community, nature, and the spiritual realm. The Navajo concept of hózhó encompasses beauty, harmony, balance, and wellness. To Walk in Beauty means to live in right relationship with all things. Disease, in this worldview, represents disharmony; something out of balance that must be restored, not simply by cutting out the offending organ but by addressing the underlying spiritual and relational imbalances [1].

Dr. Alvord began to observe that patients who underwent traditional healing ceremonies alongside Western medical treatments often did better. Navajo healers (hataali) use song, symbols (such as corn pollen, eagle feathers, masks of the Navajo gods, and sand paintings), and ceremony with their patients, and involve family and neighbors in the process. The psychological and spiritual comfort thus provided can prepare patients for surgery, childbirth, or chemotherapy, and speed their recovery afterwards [1]. She realized that the feelings and beliefs of both patient and surgeon could affect recovery time, postsurgical complications, and even survival. This wasn't mysticism; it was the mind-body connection that Western medicine was only beginning to take seriously in the 1990s, but which Native healing traditions had understood for millennia.

She started incorporating these insights into her practice. She allowed patients to bring sacred objects into the operating room. She consulted with traditional healers about timing surgeries to align with ceremonial calendars. She learned to explain Western medical procedures in terms that honored Navajo beliefs rather than dismissing them as superstition. Most importantly, she began to see her patients not as collections of organs that needed repair but as whole people embedded in complex webs of relationships and meaning [1].

This integrative approach—honoring both her Stanford surgical training and her Navajo heritage—became the defining philosophy of Dr. Alvord's career. She wrote: "Although I was a good surgeon, I was not always a good healer [7]." That distinction mattered profoundly. Surgery could fix a physical problem, but healing required addressing the whole person: body, mind, spirit, community, and environment.

In 1999, Dr. Alvord co-authored "The Scalpel and the Silver Bear: The First Navajo Woman Surgeon Combines Western Medicine and Traditional Healing," with journalist Elizabeth Cohen Van Pelt. The title itself captures the dualism at the heart of her work: the scalpel represents Western surgical precision and technology, while the silver bear—a Navajo sacred object—represents the traditional spiritual practices and beliefs of her people. The book is part memoir, part medical philosophy, and part cultural bridge-building [1, 7].

"The Scalpel and the Silver Bear," tells Dr. Alvord's remarkable journey from the reservation to Stanford and back again, but more importantly, it makes a compelling case for integrating traditional healing practices with modern medicine. She argues not that one approach is superior to the other but that they are complementary; that Western medicine's technological prowess combined with traditional medicine's holistic wisdom creates a more effective, more humane approach to healing.

The book was an immediate success, eventually selling over 50,000 copies [7, 9]. Critics praised its accessibility, wisdom, and the unique perspective it offered [7]. Tony Hillerman, the celebrated mystery writer who set many of his novels in Navajo country, wrote: "Those who enjoy an insider's look at how modern medicine and life mix with the Navajo way shouldn't miss "The Scalpel and the Silver Bear" [12]." *Publishers Weekly* called it an "inspiring memoir" that "offers intriguing ideas about humane health care [13]." The book won the Circles Book Award from

Georgia College and State University in 2000 and received the American Medical Writers Association's Award of Excellence in 1999 [9, 14].

More significantly, "The Scalpel and the Silver Bear" became required reading in medical schools and universities across the country [9]. For nearly two decades, the book has been used to teach medical students, nursing students, and healthcare professionals about cultural competency, holistic care, and the importance of understanding patients' belief systems. The book reached beyond medical education to influence broader conversations about healthcare, Native American rights, and the integration of traditional and modern healing practices.

Dr. Alvord's timing was fortuitous. The book appeared just as Western medicine was beginning to grapple seriously with questions of cultural awareness, patient-centered care, and the limits of the biomedical model. The 1990s saw growing recognition that medicine's reductionist focus on disease mechanisms had led to a crisis of meaning; physicians were technically proficient but often failed to see or treat the whole person. Alternative and complementary medicine was gaining mainstream acceptance. Mind-body medicine, once dismissed as quackery, was being validated by research on psychoneuroimmunology, the placebo effect, and the impact of stress on health outcomes.

Dr. Alvord's book provided a roadmap for how to integrate different healing traditions without abandoning scientific rigor. She didn't argue that traditional healing should replace surgery or antibiotics. She argued that ceremony, connection, and belief could enhance medical outcomes when combined with appropriate technical interventions. Her approach was pragmatic rather than ideological; whatever helped patients heal was worth considering.

The book also provided representation and inspiration for Native American students, particularly Native women considering careers in medicine or science. Here was proof that a Native woman could not only survive medical training but excel in one of its most demanding specialties while maintaining her cultural identity and values. Dr. Alvord became a role model and mentor to countless Native students navigating the often hostile terrain of academic medicine [1].

Following the success of her book, Dr. Alvord's career took on an educational and advocacy dimension alongside her surgical practice. From 1997 to 2009, she served as Associate Dean for Student Affairs and Assistant Professor of Surgery and Psychiatry at Dartmouth Medical School; returning to the institution where she had first struggled as an undergraduate, now as a leader helping to shape medical education [2, 3, 9]. She worked to recruit and support underrepresented minority students and to integrate teachings about cultural competency into the curriculum.

From 2003 onward, Dr. Alvord served as Associate Faculty at the Center for American Indian Health at Johns Hopkins School of Public Health, bringing her expertise to research and education focused on Native American health disparities. From 2008 to 2010, she served on the National Advisory Council for Complementary and Alternative Medicine (NACCAM) , advising the National Institutes of Health on research priorities and policy.

From 2010 to 2012, Dr. Alvord served as Associate Dean at the Central Michigan University College of Medicine, helping to develop a new medical school that opened in fall 2013. She played an instrumental role in shaping the curriculum and culture of this new institution. From 2012 to 2014, she was Associate Dean of Student Affairs and Admissions at the University of Arizona College of Medicine in Tucson [9].

In each of these positions, Dr. Alvord brought her unique perspective on medical education and patient care [1]. She advocated for recruiting more Native American students into medicine, for creating supportive environments where students from diverse backgrounds could thrive, and for teaching all medical students to provide culturally competent care. She pushed medical schools to accommodate religious and cultural practices; to recognize that a Navajo medical student might need time off for traditional ceremonies, or that a Muslim student's need to pray five times daily wasn't a disruption but a legitimate accommodation of faith.

In 2013, Dr. Alvord's philosophy and accomplishments earned her national recognition when both the National Indian Health Board and the National Congress of American Indians endorsed her as a candidate for Surgeon General of the United States [3, 9, 11]. While she was not ultimately appointed, the nomination itself was historic; acknowledging that a Navajo woman surgeon had insights into healthcare that the nation needed.

Dr. Alvord has received numerous other honors throughout her career. In 1992, she received the Governor's Award for Outstanding New Mexico Women from New Mexico Governor Bruce King [14, 15]. She received honorary degrees from Albany Medical College (2001), Drexel University (2006), and Pine Manor College (2009). In 2018, she received the J.E. Wallace Sterling Lifetime Achievement Award in Medicine from the Stanford Medicine Alumni Association, one of Stanford's most prestigious honors, recognizing her extraordinary contributions to medicine and medical education [11, 15].

She was featured in the National Library of Medicine exhibit "Changing the Face of Medicine" and in the PBS documentary *Medicine Woman* [1]. She has lectured widely on healing environments, Native American health, cultural competency, and the healing properties of Native American ceremonies. She has published research articles in the *Journal of the American College of Surgeons* on surgical outcomes and decision-making in American Indian and Alaska Native patients, bringing attention to healthcare disparities and the unique needs of Native populations [3].

In 2017, Dr. Alvord completed a mini-fellowship at the Cleveland Clinic, continuing her professional development even decades into her career. In 2018, she joined Astria Health in Washington State as a general surgeon, practicing at Astria Toppenish Hospital and Astria Sunnyside Hospital. She currently serves as Chief of Staff at Astria Health, where she brings over 35 years of surgical experience to a region with significant Native American and Hispanic populations and limited access to specialty care [9].

Dr. Alvord chose to practice in the Yakima Valley specifically because of the opportunity to serve underserved, rural populations, including Native Americans. "I can offer an understanding of diverse cultures and religious practices, with a personal touch," she explained. She noted that people who work in rural areas "have a sense of caring that has more depth. The care here is very good, but the caring is even better [9]."

She continues to perform the full range of general surgical procedures—gallbladder removals, hernia repairs, colonoscopies, cancer surgeries—with the same technical skill she learned at Stanford, combined with the holistic approach she learned from Navajo healers. She is Board Certified and has maintained her certification for over three decades, accepting new patients and providing compassionate, culturally informed care [9, 10].

Dr. Alvord is married to Jonathan Alvord, who is a Physician Assistant, and together they form a dedicated healthcare team serving their community. They have two children, Christopher Kodiak Alvord and Kaitlyn Arviso Alvord [10]. The family's commitment to healthcare and to serving underserved populations continues across generations.

Dr. Alvord's impact on literature and popular culture, while more modest than some of the other physician-authors in this series, is nonetheless significant. "The Scalpel and the Silver Bear," has sold steadily for over two decades and remains in print; no small feat for a nonfiction memoir. The book's use in medical schools means it has directly influenced how thousands of healthcare providers think about patient care. It has also reached general readers interested in Native American culture, women's achievements, and healthcare reform.

The book represents an important voice in Native American literature and in the medical humanities; a genre that explores the human dimensions of illness and healing through narrative. Dr. Alvord joins a small but significant group of Native American physician-writers whose work bridges cultures and challenges the dominant narratives about both Native peoples and medical care.

Perhaps most importantly, Dr. Alvord has offered a model of integration rather than assimilation. She did not abandon her Native identity to become a surgeon, nor did she reject Western medicine to remain faithful to traditional ways. Instead, she claimed both traditions, insisting that they could strengthen rather than contradict each other. Her life's work demonstrates that being deeply rooted in one's own culture can make one a better physician, not despite that rootedness but because of it.

References

1. National Library of Medicine. Biography—Dr. Lori Arviso Alvord. Changing the Face of Medicine. n.d. https://cfmedicine.nlm.nih.gov/physicians/biography_7.html.
2. Dartmouth College. Integrating healing properties of traditional Native medicine with Western practice. 2023, January 26. https://home.dartmouth.edu/events/event?event=69276.
3. Ada Lovelace Day. ALD23: Dr Lori Alvord, surgeon. 2023, October 11. https://findingada.com/blog/2023/10/11/ald23-dr-lori-alvord-surgeon/.
4. Navajo Times. First Navajo woman doctor recounts struggles in college. 2011, October 31. https://navajotimes.com/education/2011/1011/103111alvord.php.
5. Minority Business Review. Lori Arviso Alvord (Navajo Nation). 2023, December 22. https://minoritybusinessreview.com/lori-arviso-alvord-navajo-nation/.

6. Stanford University Medical Center, 25 years. Stanford Medicine, 2(1, Suppl.), XX. 1984, Fall.
7. Alvord LA, Van Pelt EC. The scalpel and the silver bear: the first Navajo woman surgeon combines Western medicine and traditional healing. Des Plaines: Bantam Books; 1999.
8. Kirkus Reviews. The scalpel and the silver bear. n.d. https://www.kirkusreviews.com/book-reviews/md-alvord/the-scalpel-and-the-silver-bear/.
9. Astria Health. Lori Alvord, MD. n.d. https://www.astria.health/provider-directory/provider/lori-alvord.
10. Stanford Magazine. Through Navajo eyes. 2000, January/February. https://stanfordmag.org/contents/through-navajo-eyes.
11. Association of American Indian Physicians. Dr. Lori Arviso Alvord being honored with J.E. Wallace Sterling Lifetime Achievement Award in Medicine. n.d. https://www.aaip.org/news/dr-lori-arviso-alvord-being-honored-with-j-e-wallace-sterling-lifetime-achievement-award-in-medicine.
12. Amazon. The scalpel and the silver bear: the first Navajo woman surgeon combines Western medicine and traditional healing. n.d. https://www.amazon.com/Scalpel-Silver-Bear-Combines-Traditional/dp/0553378007.
13. Publishers Weekly. The scalpel and the silver bear. 1999. http://www.publishersweekly.com/9780553100129.
14. University of Wisconsin Interfaces. Lori Alvord. n.d. https://interfaces.che.wisc.edu/lori-alvord/.
15. Astria Health. Stanford University honors Astria Health general surgeon, Lori Arviso Alvord, MD. 2018, December 3. https://www.astria.health/news/stanford-university-honors-astria-health-general-surgeon-lori-arviso-alvord-md.

Chapter 16
Pauline Chen, MD

The large majority of medical training is focused on identifying the various methods by which we might prolong patient lives, with a portion of training devoted to optimizing quality of life to align with patient goals and a sliver allocated to navigating end-of-life care. Arguably each person's last moment is unique, and preparedness for that variation is challenging within a fixed time frame of formal education. However, much like we were given the opportunity to practice our clinical techniques and history gathering acumen, with so-called "standardized patients," there should be time dedicated to understanding how to approach death. And not simply for the sake of appropriately delivering bad news, but as a protective mechanism for those who will necessarily meet with death in our clinics, in our wards, in our nurseries and in our ICUs. There is no perfect shield that will blunt the ache of losing a patient, but there is disservice in not discussing this near inevitability. While I called upon the correct words to explain the end of a son to his father, I struggled with the internal monologue necessary to resume the rest of my 28-h call. Reading Dr. Chen's words in "Final Exam," was a reminder that this need not be a solitary struggle, and that we all could use the CME in approaching death amongst our patients.

Dr. Pauline Chen was born in 1964 to Taiwanese immigrant parents [1–3] who, like so many families arriving on American shores, carried with them dreams of educational opportunity and professional advancement. The trajectory of her life would eventually lead her to the pinnacles of academic medicine, but perhaps more importantly, to a reckoning with medicine's most profound failure: its inability to meaningfully prepare patients, families, and physicians themselves for death. Her journey from the elite halls of Harvard University through the rigorous gauntlet of surgical training would ultimately produce not just a technically skilled transplant surgeon, but a physician-writer who dared to articulate what many in medicine feel but few have the courage to voice.

Dr. Chen's educational pedigree reads like a roadmap through America's most prestigious institutions. After graduating from The Loomis Chaffee School, she attended Harvard University before pursuing her medical degree at Northwestern

O. M. Cox, *The Pen, The Stethoscope, and The Scalpel*, https://doi.org/10.1007/978-3-032-19406-0_16

University's Feinberg School of Medicine [1–3]. Her surgical training took her through Yale University, the National Cancer Institute at the National Institutes of Health, and finally to UCLA, where she would eventually join the faculty specializing in liver and kidney transplants and cancer treatment [1, 4, 5]. This path through academic medicine's most respected programs might suggest a conventional narrative of success, but Dr. Chen's story would prove to be anything but conventional.

It was during these years of training that Dr. Chen began to notice a disturbing pattern, one that would eventually become the central thesis of her literary work. Despite being surrounded by death on a daily basis, despite witnessing countless patients transition from life to its inevitable conclusion, the medical establishment seemed fundamentally unprepared to discuss, much less guide, this universal human experience [6]. The hidden curriculum of medical education, as she would later term it, taught young physicians to view death as failure, to close the curtain around dying patients and their families, to focus on the next operative case rather than sit with those facing mortality.

The transformation from surgeon to writer began not with a deliberate plan but with a haunting. Dr. Chen speaks of a young patient, a favorite, whom she abandoned to painful and futile end-of-life care because she could not bear to see him diminished by cancer. In the idiom of her Taiwanese heritage, he became a *wan ong kuei*, a restless soul who would not leave her in peace [4, 7]. Five years later, pregnant with twins and taking time off from her work as a transplant surgeon at UCLA, Dr. Chen finally confronted this ghost. The result was "Final Exam: A Surgeon's Reflections on Mortality," published by Alfred A. Knopf in 2007.

"Final Exam" stands as Dr. Chen's most significant contribution to medical literature, and it remains her only full-length book, though its impact has reverberated far beyond what a single volume might ordinarily achieve. The book became a *New York Times* bestseller and has been translated into nearly a dozen languages, reaching audiences across the world who recognized in Dr. Chen's words their own struggles with mortality, whether as physicians, patients, or family members [1, 7, 8]. It was named a finalist for the Books for a Better Life Award and recognized by the *New York Times* book critics as one of the ten best books published that year.

The power of "Final Exam," lies in its unrelenting honesty and its narrative structure. Rather than approaching the subject of medical education and death through abstract analysis or policy recommendations, Dr. Chen chose to tell stories. She begins at the beginning, with the moment every medical student remembers with crystalline clarity: the unveiling of the cadaver that will be their first patient. Through this lens, she traces her journey through medical school at Northwestern and residency at Yale, documenting the gradual process by which empathetic young people enter medicine with idealistic dreams of healing and emerge as technically proficient but emotionally distant physicians [4, 7].

The *New York Times* reviewer noted that "the real power of her book lies in her stories. Balanced and perfect, each one seeks out the reader's heart like a guided missile, and explodes [9]." This assessment captures the essence of Dr. Chen's literary approach. She does not lecture; she bears witness. She recounts the patient whose cholangiocarcinoma led to a choice between dying in the ICU under aggressive intervention or going home with palliative care. She describes her own evolution from a resident who would avoid dying patients to a surgeon who finally understood that presence itself constitutes care, that comfort and the alleviation of suffering represent medicine's highest calling even when cure proves impossible.

Dr. Atul Gawande, a physician-writer of considerable acclaim and author of "Being Mortal," wrote of "Final Exam": "This is a revealing and heartfelt book. Pauline Chen takes us where few do, inside the feeling of practicing surgery, with its doubts, failures, and triumphs. Her tales are also uncommonly moving, most especially when contemplating death and our difficulties as doctors and patients in coming to grips with it [1, 7]." The endorsement from Dr. Gawande, who would later write extensively on similar themes, underscores Dr. Chen's pioneering role in bringing these conversations into mainstream medical discourse.

The critical reception of "Final Exam," highlighted Dr. Chen's prose style, which reviewers consistently described as graceful, lucid, and precise. The *San Francisco Chronicle* noted that "Chen has a clear and unwavering eye for exposing the reality behind the mythology of medical training. We would all do well to listen to what she has to say [7]." The *Los Angeles Times Book Review* praised the work as "fresh and honest," while *Publishers Weekly* commended her "immaculately honed prose and moral passion [1, 7, 10]." These assessments recognize not just the importance of Dr. Chen's subject matter but her skill as a literary craftsperson, her ability to wield language with the same precision she once brought to the operating room.

What distinguishes Dr. Chen's writing from other physician memoirs is her willingness to interrogate her own failures with the same rigor she applies to systemic problems in medical education. She does not position herself as having achieved an epiphany or as offering easy solutions. Instead, she documents her ongoing struggle to reconcile technical excellence with human compassion, to maintain her capacity for empathy in a profession that systematically erodes it. In one particularly powerful passage, she describes pronouncing a patient dead for the first time, the weight of those words, the ritual of checking for absent vital signs while the body still held warmth. She captures the paradox of becoming increasingly familiar with death while simultaneously growing more uncomfortable with it, more invested in avoiding it at all costs.

The book's final scene offers a moment of transformation, though Dr. Chen characteristically refuses to present it as complete or permanent. A patient with cholangiocarcinoma chooses to die at home rather than pursue futile aggressive treatment. Dr. Chen supports this decision, accompanies the patient and family through the process, provides comfort rather than false hope. Yet even in this moment of apparent growth, she acknowledges her continued struggle. Speaking with grieving family members, she begins with her usual refrain: "I wish I could have cured him, I wish I could have done more." But then comes the realization, the insight that feels hard-won rather than easily achieved: "It was then I realized that I had done more. I had comforted my patient and his family. I had eased their suffering; I had been present for them during life and despite death."

This conclusion, with its qualified optimism and honest acknowledgment of ongoing struggle, exemplifies Dr. Chen's literary approach. She offers no simple redemption narrative, no suggestion that reading the right book or attending the right conference will solve medicine's dysfunctional relationship with death. Instead, she suggests that awareness itself, the willingness to examine our failures and discomforts, represents the beginning of change.

Following the success of "Final Exam," Dr. Chen expanded her platform by launching "Doctor and Patient," a regular online column for the *New York Times* [11]. This body of work, spanning several years and dozens of essays, allowed Dr. Chen to address a broader range of issues affecting the physician-patient relationship while maintaining her focus on the human dimensions of medical practice. The column covered topics from hand hygiene compliance to moral distress among healthcare workers, from the role of nurses in patient care to the challenges of medical education reform. Through this platform, Dr. Chen reached millions of readers, many of them outside the medical profession, bringing insider perspectives on healthcare to a general audience hungry for such insights.

The "Doctor and Patient" column demonstrated Dr. Chen's ability to synthesize personal experience, medical literature, and broader cultural analysis. She interviewed researchers, cited studies, and incorporated diverse voices while always grounding her writing in concrete stories and specific moments of clinical care. A piece on compassion fatigue among nurses, for instance, began with a portrait of a senior nurse who injured her back, then expanded to discuss the systemic factors contributing to healthcare worker burnout and the economic costs of failing to address these issues. Throughout, Dr. Chen maintained the respectful, nuanced tone that characterized "Final Exam," avoiding easy condemnation while clearly articulating the stakes involved.

The column also revealed Dr. Chen's growing interest in the broader infrastructure of healthcare delivery. She wrote about accountable care organizations, patient satisfaction surveys, and the economic pressures shaping clinical decision-making. Yet even in these pieces, which might easily have become dry policy discussions, Dr. Chen centered human experience. When writing about cost-cutting pressures, she described a patient who could barely afford prescribed dressing supplies, using this encounter to explore the gap between clinical training and the socioeconomic realities that profoundly affect health outcomes. This approach made abstract policy debates concrete and urgent, demonstrating the real-world consequences of systemic choices.

Dr. Chen's impact on medicine extends beyond her published work. She became a sought-after speaker at medical schools, hospitals, palliative care organizations, and bioethics conferences across the country and internationally. Institutions from the Association of American Medical Colleges to the National Hospice and Palliative Care Organization to TED Global invited her to address their audiences. Those who heard her speak consistently remarked on the power of her presentations, which, like her writing, combined personal narrative with broader insights about healthcare delivery and medical education [9, 12].

The awards she accumulated testify to her peers' recognition of her contributions. In 1999, while still primarily focused on clinical work, she received the UCLA Outstanding Physician of the Year Award [1, 13]. Earlier, during her training at Yale, she was honored with the George Longstreth Humanness Award, given to the trainee who most exemplifies "empathy, kindness, and care in an age of advancing technology [1, 9, 13]." This latter award takes on additional poignancy when considered alongside Dr. Chen's later writing about how surgical training systematically erodes these very qualities. The Chinese American Medical Society recognized her work with their Distinguished Community Service Award, while the Association of Women Surgeons presented her with the Olga Jonasson Distinguished Member Award [14].

As a writer, Dr. Chen's work earned recognition beyond the medical community. Her essay "Dead Enough? The Paradox of Brain Death," published in *The Virginia Quarterly Review* in 2005, was a finalist for a 2006 National Magazine Award. She was the 2005 co-winner of the Staige D. Blackford Prize for Nonfiction and a finalist for the 2002 James Kirkwood Prize in Creative Writing. These honors from the literary establishment validated Dr. Chen's dual identity as physician and writer, demonstrating that her work achieved not just medical relevance but literary excellence.

The trajectory of Dr. Chen's career represents an increasingly common pattern among physician-writers: the gradual shift from full-time clinical practice to a hybrid role emphasizing writing, teaching, and advocacy. By the time her twins were born and "Final Exam" was published, Dr. Chen had begun transitioning away from the demanding schedule of transplant surgery. She eventually worked at the West Roxbury Veterans Administration Hospital while devoting more time to writing and speaking. According to her publisher, she lives near Boston with her husband and children, continuing to write and lecture on healthcare issues while maintaining some clinical work [15].

This evolution from surgeon to writer should not be read as an abandonment of medicine but rather as an expansion of how Dr. Chen chose to serve the profession and its patients. Through her writing and speaking, she reached far more healthcare workers and patients than she ever could have treated individually in the operating room. Her work influenced medical school curricula, inspired conversations about end-of-life care reform, and validated the experiences of countless physicians who felt the same discomfort with death that Dr. Chen so eloquently articulated.

The cultural impact of Chen's work lies primarily in its timing and accessibility. She published "Final Exam" at a moment when conversations about end-of-life care were beginning to enter mainstream discourse, but when physician voices on these topics remained relatively rare. Earlier physician-writers like Dr. Elisabeth Kübler-Ross had addressed death and dying, but primarily from psychiatry or palliative care perspectives. Dr. Chen wrote as a surgeon, someone trained in the most interventionist specialty, whose entire professional identity centered on aggressive action to preserve life. Her willingness to question this paradigm, to suggest that surgical skill might sometimes cause harm rather than good when applied to dying patients, carried particular weight.

Moreover, Dr. Chen's platform at the *New York Times* gave her access to a readership far broader than most medical writing achieves. Millions of people who would never pick up a medical journal or attend a medical conference encountered her ideas through the newspaper. Patients and families grappling with end-of-life decisions found in her work both validation and guidance. Healthcare administrators and policymakers gained insight into the human costs of systemic failures. Medical students and residents discovered that their struggles with death were not personal failings but predictable consequences of how medicine trains its practitioners.

Dr. Chen argues, through both direct statement and implication, that medicine's approach to death harms everyone involved. Patients die in ICUs undergoing painful interventions when they would have chosen comfort care had the option been presented clearly. Families face complicated grief, wondering whether they advocated effectively for their loved ones, haunted by the violence of aggressive end-of-life treatment. Physicians experience burnout, moral distress, and compassion fatigue, their idealism ground down by the constant demand to attempt the impossible while pretending death represents failure rather than inevitability. The system itself bleeds resources, devoting extraordinary expenses to treatments that prolong suffering rather than life.

Yet "Final Exam" is not fundamentally a book of critique or complaint. Instead, it functions as witness and invitation. Dr. Chen bears witness to the costs of medicine's denial of death, but she also documents moments of grace, instances when physicians do manage to provide meaningful comfort and guidance to dying patients and their families. She invites readers, particularly physician readers, to examine their own practices and assumptions, to consider whether the technical excellence we pursue might sometimes obscure more fundamental obligations to our patients.

The question Dr. Chen poses at the opening of "Final Exam" deserves repetition: "Why are we so bad at taking care of the dying?" Her answer, developed over more than 200 pages of memoir and analysis, points to multiple interconnected factors. Medical education systematically teaches depersonalization as a survival mechanism, helping students and residents function despite constant exposure to suffering and death. Professional culture equates death with failure, making physicians reluctant to acknowledge when cure becomes impossible. The scientific foundation of modern medicine privileges measurable interventions over less tangible forms of care like presence and comfort. Economic incentives reward aggressive treatment over palliative approaches. Legal fears make physicians hesitant to stop treatments once started. And perhaps most fundamentally, our broader cultural denial of death's inevitability finds its most concentrated expression in medical settings, where technological capability creates an illusion of control over mortality itself.

For those of us navigating medical training and early practice, Dr. Chen's writing offers several forms of value. Most immediately, it provides validation that the discomfort and distress we feel when patients die represents not personal inadequacy but a natural response to genuinely difficult experiences. Dr. Pauline Chen, through one remarkable book and a body of complementary writing, gave medicine a mirror in which to examine its relationship with mortality and a map toward more humane alternatives. The profession has yet to fully embrace the changes her work implies, but her voice continues to call us toward our better selves, toward the physicians we hoped to become when we first entered medical school with dreams of healing.

References

1. Penguin Random House. Pauline W. Chen. n.d. https://www.penguinrandomhouse.com/authors/74324/pauline-w-chen/.
2. The Loomis Chaffee School. Pauline Chen '82, trustee and chair of the Diversity Task Force. n.d. https://www.loomischaffee.org/cf_news/view.cfm?newsid=4026.
3. Thompson B. Cutting to the core. The Washington Post. 2007, January 29. https://www.washingtonpost.com/archive/lifestyle/2007/01/29/cutting-to-the-core-span-classbankheadsurgeons-are-taught-to-view-death-coldly/2eaee71b-cc14-4379-a253-e998bab8c028/.
4. Chen PW. Final exam: a surgeon's reflections on mortality. New York: Alfred A. Knopf; 2007.
5. UCLA Health. Past fellows. 2015. https://www.uclahealth.org/departments/surgery/education/fellowships/abdominal-transplant-hepatobiliary-surgery/past-fellows.
6. Mehegan D. The doctor and death. The Boston Globe. 2007. https://www.hospicevolunteerassociation.org/HVANewsletter/0090_Vol3No2_2007Mar27_TheDoctorAndDeath.pdf.
7. Amazon. Final Exam: a surgeon's reflections on mortality. n.d. https://www.amazon.com/Final-Exam-Surgeons-Reflections-Mortality/dp/030727537X.
8. New Jersey Health Care Quality Institute (NJHCQI). Pauline Chen. n.d. https://www.njhcqi.org/medicaid-policy-center-old/paulinechen/.
9. PRH Speakers Bureau. Pauline Chen, M.D.: Healthcare & medicine author, speaker. n.d. https://www.prhspeakers.com/speaker/pauline-chen.
10. Publishers Weekly. Final Exam: a surgeon's reflections on mortality. 2007. http://www.publishersweekly.com/9780307263537.
11. Chen PW. Doctor and patient. The New York Times. n.d. https://archive.nytimes.com/well.blogs.nytimes.com/author/pauline-w-chen-md/.
12. Harvard University Ackerman Symposium. Self & non-self: a transplant surgeon and the medical humanities. n.d. https://ackerman.harvard.edu/event/2008-ackerman-symposium-medicine-and-culture-self-non-self-transplant-surgeon.
13. Virginia Quarterly Review. Pauline W. Chen. n.d. https://www.vqronline.org/people/pauline-w-chen.
14. Bulletin of the American College of Surgeons. Dr. Chen delivering the Olga Jonasson Lecture [Photograph]. 2014, January. https://bulletin.facs.org/2014/01/highlights-of-the-2013-clinical-congress/cc-2013-pauline-chen-delivering-olga-jonasson-lecture-dsc_6192/.
15. Inzone P. Dr. Pauline W. Chen '82 to speak at Commencement. The Loomis Chaffee Log. 2020. https://lc-log.org/wp-content/uploads/2020/05/Log-Commencement-2020-final-compressed.pdf.

Chapter 17
Sayantani DasGupta, MD

I grew up in a house full of avid readers, from my mother, whose shelves were a blend of romance and mystery, to my father who engrossed himself in autobiographies and to my sister, who wrote young adult fiction in her spare time, while drawing inspiration from Ann M. Martin. My catalog of completed literary fiction numbered in the thousands by the time I hit puberty. For both my sister and I, having a book in tow, at all times was critical to our peace of mind. No matter the occasion, the ability to dive headfirst into a new world at the flip of a page was irresistible. I had explored every realm from Tortall to Narnia to Middle Earth, absorbed myself in the universes of Nancy Drew, Goosebumps, and The Baby-Sitters Club, and could spot the signatures of authors like Enid Blyton, Francine Pascal and Judy Blume, scrawled across book spines from a mile away. And yet, while I simply inserted myself into these stories, a willing ally or protagonist within the world, their covers were a constant reminder that I was not centered in their sphere. As an adolescent, I never spent much time investigating my belonging in these fictional spaces; my imagination was sufficient to cover the entrance fee. As an adult, I recognize the power of being a described principal lead, even in fiction, to support healthy maturation and self-realization. Nowadays, I find there is significantly more variety in main characters, as authors from minoritized groups in the United States have enriched the temples of fantasy, science fiction, mystery, romance and historical fiction, with characters who look and sound like the global majority. Dr. Sayantani DasGupta is one of such authors, whose unique insight into children, as a pediatrician, informs the brilliant, engaging heroes she creates.

Dr. Sayantani DasGupta was born in 1970 in Columbus, Ohio, to Sujan and Shamita Das DasGupta, Bengali immigrants who came to the United States carrying not just hopes for their own futures but also the weight of a family history steeped in political activism and resistance [1]. Her mother, Shamita Das DasGupta, would become a renowned activist, scholar, and co-founder of Manavi, one of the first organizations in the United States to address domestic violence within the South Asian community [2, 3]. This lineage of advocacy, resistance, and storytelling

O. M. Cox, *The Pen, The Stethoscope, and The Scalpel*,
https://doi.org/10.1007/978-3-032-19406-0_17

would profoundly shape Sayantani's approach to both medicine and literature, informing her understanding that narratives possess healing power and that centering marginalized voices constitutes a form of justice [4].

Growing up between Ohio and New Jersey, a younger Sayantani heard bedtime stories vastly different from those filling the shelves of her local library [3]. While her classmates learned of Cinderella and Snow White, her parents regaled her with tales of brave princesses, bloodthirsty rakkhosh demons, and flying pakkhiraj horses [1, 5, 6]. These Bengali folktales, passed down through generations, existed in sharp contrast to the literature she encountered in school, where brown-skinned protagonists were conspicuously absent and South Asian characters, when they appeared at all, were relegated to stereotypical roles or cautionary narratives about "backward" cultures needing Western salvation [1, 5]. This disconnect between the rich, powerful stories of her heritage and the limited, often demeaning representations in mainstream media would later fuel her commitment to creating children's literature that centers joy, agency, and adventure for characters of color [1].

Dr. DasGupta's academic trajectory took her through some of America's most prestigious institutions [4]. She completed her undergraduate education at Brown University before pursuing her medical degree and Master of Public Health at Johns Hopkins University, graduating in 1998 [1, 4]. Her memoir of medical school, "Her Own Medicine: A Woman's Journey from Student to Doctor," published by Ballantine Books in 1999, emerged from what she termed her "field notes;" observations she recorded throughout her training as a means of surviving the experience [1, 7, 8]. The book offers a raw examination of medical education's hierarchical structure, its gender dynamics, and what she identified as medicine's troubling militaristic culture where patients could become positioned as enemies rather than people deserving care and compassion.

In "Her Own Medicine,","Dr. DasGupta describes entering medical school with idealistic visions of saving lives and creating positive change, only to encounter a rigid, often hostile environment marked by hierarchies, gender discrimination, and systematic dehumanization of both patients and trainees [7, 8]. The book illuminates her experiences through vivid patient stories—a 14-year-old giving birth, terrified AIDS patients, elderly patients with complex needs—while critiquing the structural problems of managed care, the gender wars within medicine, and what she termed the "militarism of medicine." Critics noted both the book's political engagement and its literary quality, praising Dr. DasGupta's ability to blend personal narrative with systemic critique [7, 8]. Though some reviewers found its focus on institutional critique rather than personal anecdote limiting, the memoir established Dr. DasGupta as a physician-writer unafraid to name medicine's failures and imagine alternatives.

Following medical school, Dr. DasGupta completed her residency in the Social Pediatrics program at Montefiore Hospital in the Bronx, affiliated with Albert Einstein College of Medicine [1, 6–8]. It was during this period, practicing as a pediatrician in the late 1990s and early 2000s, that she began to sense both the potential and the limitations of her training. She could diagnose conditions, prescribe treatments, follow protocols with technical proficiency. Yet when patients shared their stories—narratives of illness interwoven with experiences of racism, poverty, immigration, cultural dislocation—she felt she lacked the tools to truly hear, interpret, and respond with the depth and dignity these stories deserved. Medical school had trained her rigorously in hard sciences but had largely neglected the humanities, leaving her narratively competent by accident of personal inclination rather than by design of educational curriculum.

This realization led Dr. DasGupta to a pivotal encounter that would reshape her career. In 2001, newly arrived at Columbia University, she knocked on the door of Dr. Rita Charon, a colleague she had heard was doing innovative work at the intersection of medicine and the humanities [9]. Dr. Charon, a practicing internist who had also earned a PhD in English literature, had secured a grant from the National Institutes of Health to explore how narrative skills might enhance medical practice [10, 11]. She had gathered an interdisciplinary team of scholars from philosophy, English, comparative literature, medical anthropology, and creative writing to co-create what would become known as narrative medicine.

Dr. DasGupta joined this founding group, becoming a faculty founder of what would evolve into Columbia's Master's Program in Narrative Medicine [4, 12]. The field emerged from a simple but radical premise: that caring for the sick requires not just biomedical knowledge but also narrative competence; the ability to elicit, interpret, and act upon the stories patients tell about their experiences of illness, suffering, and healing. As Dr. DasGupta would later write, "You'd better be good at pharmacology, you'd better be good at physiology, you need to know your organ systems, and you need to know how to elicit and attend to stories [1]." This attention to narrative, she argued, was not supplementary to good medicine but intrinsic to it, particularly in addressing health disparities and promoting social justice.

Within narrative medicine, Dr. DasGupta developed several key concepts that have influenced how clinicians approach patient care. Most notable is her articulation of "narrative humility," which she describes as an acknowledgment "that stories are not objects we can comprehend or ever become 100% competent regarding, particularly when those stories are oral interchanges with real live people on the other end [13, 14]." This stance contrasts with the more common medical goal of achieving narrative "competence," suggesting instead that clinicians should approach patients as teachers, recognizing themselves as lifelong learners who must continuously practice listening to and surrendering to the other. Drawing on Buddhist philosophy and oral history methodologies, narrative humility emphasizes the nonjudgmental acceptance of patient testimony and the recognition that some dimensions of another person's experience will always exceed our understanding [13, 14].

Dr. DasGupta's scholarly contributions to narrative medicine have appeared in prestigious journals including *The Lancet*, *JAMA*, *Pediatrics*, *The Hastings Center Report*, *Literature and Medicine*, and *The Journal of Medical Humanities* [12, 15]. She serves as associate editor of *Literature and Medicine* and co-authored *The Principles and Practice of Narrative Medicine* (Oxford University Press, 2017) with Dr. Rita Charon and other founding members of the Columbia program [4, 12]. This comprehensive text, which won the Perkins Award for Narrative, synthesizes over a decade of research, education, and clinical practice, offering both theoretical grounding and practical methods for implementing narrative medicine in diverse healthcare settings [16]. The book articulates six core tenets of the field: attention, representation, affiliation, action toward social justice, inclusivity, and tolerating ambiguity.

Beyond this foundational text, Dr. DasGupta has co-edited important collections that expand the boundaries of medical humanities. "Stories of Illness and Healing: Women Write their Bodies" (Kent State University Press, 2007), co-edited with Marsha Hurst, won the Silver Medal in the Women's Issues category of the Independent Publisher Book Awards and was a finalist for the ForeWord Magazine Book of the Year Award [12]. This anthology centers women's first-person narratives of illness, disability, and healing, giving voice to experiences often marginalized in mainstream medical discourse. Later, Dr. DasGupta co-edited "Globalization and Transnational Surrogacy in India: Outsourcing Life" (Lexington Books, 2014), examining the complex ethical, social, and health implications of commercial surrogacy through interdisciplinary lenses [12, 15].

At Columbia, Dr. DasGupta teaches in multiple programs and departments, reflecting her interdisciplinary approach to knowledge production. She holds positions in the Master's Program in Narrative Medicine, the Center for the Study of Ethnicity and Race, and the Institute for Comparative Literature and Society [1, 4]. She also advises in Columbia's undergraduate major in medical humanities and co-chairs the University Seminar in Narrative, Health and Social Justice [14]. Additionally, she teaches in the Health Advocacy graduate program at Sarah Lawrence College, training future advocates to understand and interpret personal, communal, and institutional narratives [4, 17]. She is a faculty founder of Columbia's provost-funded Pedagogy of Listening Lab, which explores listening as both skill and ethical practice. Her current scholarly interests focus on narrative humility in medical education and practice, racial justice and health, diaspora studies, and what she terms "science fiction/health futurities;" explorations of how speculative fiction can help us imagine more just health futures [4].

Yet as remarkable as Dr. DasGupta's contributions to academic medicine and medical humanities have been, her impact on children's literature may ultimately reach even more people and prove equally transformative. Her path to becoming a New York Times bestselling children's author began with her mother, with whom she co-authored "The Demon Slayers and Other Stories: Bengali Folktales" (Interlink, 1995) [1, 15]. This early collaboration established a pattern that would characterize her literary work: drawing on her cultural heritage to create stories that center South Asian characters, mythologies, and experiences while making them accessible to all readers. The book honored the oral storytelling traditions that had shaped her own childhood, preserving them for new generations while also making them available to children who, like her younger self, rarely saw their cultures reflected in library shelves.

For years, Dr. DasGupta continued her dual career as pediatrician and narrative medicine scholar while nurturing her fiction writing. She attended writing conferences, took classes, read widely in children's literature, and joined critique groups of fellow writers. In 2011, she attempted to publish a fantasy adventure novel featuring a Bengali American protagonist, and faced rejection after rejection. The U.S. children's book market, it seemed, was not ready for what she offered: a funny, intergalactic, fantasy adventure starring a brown-skinned Bengali immigrant daughter living in New Jersey. Rather than abandon the project, Dr. DasGupta continued revising, improving her craft, waiting for the market and her manuscript to align.

That alignment finally came in February 2018 with the publication of "The Serpent's Secret," the first book in the Kiranmala and the Kingdom Beyond series [1, 18]. The novel introduces 12-year-old Kiranmala, who lives in Parsippany, New Jersey, and believes herself to be an ordinary sixth-grader until her parents mysteriously vanish and a rakkhosh demon crashes through her kitchen intent on eating her. It turns out her parents' bedtime stories were true: she is an Indian princess from another dimension called the Kingdom Beyond, and she must undertake a dangerous quest to save her parents and prevent the evil Serpent King from collapsing all the stories of the universe into one authoritarian narrative.

"The Serpent's Secret" achieved both critical acclaim and commercial success, entering the *New York Times* bestseller list and collecting honors including Bank Street Best Book of the Year, a Booklist Best Middle Grade Novel of the twenty-first century, and an E.B. White Read Aloud Honor Book [1, 19]. The National Science Teachers Association named it an Outstanding Trade Science Book for incorporating string theory and other scientific concepts into its fantastical narrative [12]. Reviewers and readers praised Dr. DasGupta's ability to blend Bengali folktales with contemporary science, to create a protagonist who was brave, funny, and deeply relatable regardless of readers' own cultural backgrounds, and to craft an adventure story that centered joy and agency rather than trauma [1, 18].

The series continued with "Game of Stars" (2019) and "The Chaos Curse" (2020) [12, 20], each building on the world-building and character development of its predecessor while exploring themes of narrative power, authoritarian control of stories, friendship, family, and the importance of maintaining multiple, diverse narratives rather than collapsing into a single, dominant story. The books draw explicit parallels between the Serpent King's desire to control all narratives and real-world attempts to suppress diverse voices, to ban books, to insist on singular versions of history and identity. Through Kiranmala's adventures, young readers encounter ideas about representation, resistance, and the power of storytelling that resonate far beyond the fantasy genre.

What makes the Kiranmala series particularly significant is how it addresses representation without making representation itself the plot. Kiranmala is a Bengali American protagonist, yes, and the books celebrate Bengali culture through food, language, mythology, and family dynamics. But the story is not about her being Bengali American, it's an adventure about saving the multiverse. This distinction matters enormously. As Dr. DasGupta has noted in interviews and essays, there exists a troubling pattern in children's publishing where stories featuring protagonists of color are expected to center trauma, to educate white readers about racism or cultural difference, to position brown and Black children as objects of pity requiring rescue. Such narratives, even when well-intentioned, can reinforce stereotypes and deny children of color the same access to joy, adventure, and power that white characters routinely enjoy.

In an essay titled "No More Sad Brown Girls: Why Joy Is Resistance In Asian American Children's Stories," Dr. DasGupta articulates this critique forcefully [5, 21]. She describes how even today, when publishing has made some progress toward diversity, there remains a bias toward privileging stories of suffering over stories of joy when it comes to characters of color. Drawing on scholar Gayatri Chakravorty Spivak's analysis of the colonial trope of "white men saving brown women from brown men," she notes how Western fascination with brown women's pain functions to evoke saviorism while reinforcing stereotypes about "backward" or "oppressive" communities. When children's literature consistently shows brown girls crying, suffering, needing rescue, it tells both brown children and white children powerful messages about whose lives matter, whose pain is centered, whose joy is celebrated.

Against this pattern, Dr. DasGupta consciously creates stories where South Asian characters get to be powerful, funny, beloved by supportive families and communities, capable of changing the world. When Kiranmala wears kurtas with purple combat boots, when she banters with princes and battles demons, when she uses her intelligence and courage to solve interdimensional problems, she offers readers—particularly South Asian readers—a vision of themselves as heroes, not victims. As Dr. DasGupta writes, "When the world wants to see brown girls crying, our joy can be a form of important resistance [21]."

Beyond the Kiranmala series, Dr. DasGupta has expanded the Kingdom Beyond multiverse through additional series and stand-alone novels. The Fire Queen series, beginning with "Force of Fire" (2021) and continuing with "Crown of Flames," shifts focus to Pinki, a rakkhosh (demon) who must embrace her identity to serve the greater good, offering an explicitly anticolonial narrative about resistance, interspecies relationships, and challenging systems of oppression [12, 22]. The Secrets of the Sky trilogy takes an environmentally themed approach to adventures in the same universe. She has also written "She Persisted: Virginia Apgar" (2021) as part of Chelsea Clinton's *She Persisted* series, profiling the physician who created the Apgar Score for assessing newborn health; a choice that connects her children's writing back to medicine while highlighting a woman in science [12].

More recently, Dr. DasGupta has ventured into young adult contemporary fiction with Jane Austen-inspired retellings. "Debating Darcy" (2022) reimagines "Pride and Prejudice," while "Rosewood: A Midsummer Meet Cute" (2023) draws on "Sense and Sensibility [12, 19]." These novels demonstrate her range as a writer, her ability to honor classic literature while updating it for contemporary, diverse audiences. Her forthcoming novel "Theft of the Ruby Lotus" promises a museum heist and art repatriation adventure, addressing questions of colonial looting and cultural property with the same commitment to centering South Asian perspectives and protagonists.

In total, Dr. DasGupta has authored or co-authored over fifteen books spanning academic medicine, medical humanities, memoir, folktales, middle-grade fantasy, and young adult contemporary fiction [12]. This remarkable productivity across genres reflects her fundamental understanding that stories, in all their forms, constitute "good medicine," a phrase she uses repeatedly to describe narrative's healing power. Whether writing scholarly articles about narrative humility for physicians-in-training, co-editing collections of women's illness narratives, or creating fantasy adventures for middle-schoolers, Dr. DasGupta pursues a consistent project: honoring stories, centering marginalized voices, and recognizing that who gets to tell which stories shapes possibilities for healing, justice, and flourishing.

Dr. DasGupta's impact on children's literature extends beyond her own writing through her work with We Need Diverse Books (WNDB), where she serves as a team member involved in social media outreach and advocacy [19, 23]. WNDB emerged in 2014 as a grassroots organization advocating for essential changes in the publishing industry to produce and promote literature that reflects and honors the lives of all young people. The organization provides grants to writers and illustrators from marginalized backgrounds, offers mentorship programs, advocates against book bans, and works to increase diversity among publishing professionals. Dr. DasGupta's involvement reflects her commitment to systemic change; she recognizes that individual books, however excellent, cannot alone transform a publishing landscape that has historically excluded, exoticized, or misrepresented communities of color.

Through WNDB and in her own advocacy, Dr. DasGupta addresses what she terms the "chai-latte-fication" of South Asian identities in children's literature [24]. This phrase captures how mainstream publishing tends to reduce the rich diversity of South Asian cultures—myriad ethnicities, religions, languages, mythologies, foods, and tradition—to a narrow set of recognizable signifiers: Bollywood, samosas, sarees, chai. Indian and Indian American narratives dominate South Asian representation because they align with Western audiences' existing (limited) knowledge, while Sri Lankan, Pakistani, Bangladeshi, Nepali, Bhutanese, and Maldivian stories remain largely invisible. Even within Indian representation, North Indian Hindu experiences often stand in for all South Asian experiences, erasing the specificity of Bengali, Tamil, Telugu, Malayali, and countless other distinct cultures.

As a Bengali American writer, Dr. DasGupta resists this homogenization through careful attention to cultural specificity. She spells words "the Bengali way rather than the Hindi way," includes Bengali-specific cultural references, jokes, and practices, and centers her characters' particular regional and religious identities rather than defaulting to generic "South Asian" representation. This specificity serves multiple purposes: it honors the actual diversity within South Asian communities, it gives Bengali American readers the experience of seeing their specific culture centered, and it educates all readers that "South Asian" encompasses multitudes. Yet she accomplishes this cultural grounding while keeping her stories accessible to readers unfamiliar with Bengali culture, through context clues, warm humor, and universal themes of friendship, family, courage, and belonging.

The cover of "The Serpent's Secret" illustrates her collaborative approach to representation. Dr. DasGupta worked closely with Scholastic's art director Elizabeth Parisi and illustrator Vivienne To, serving as what she terms a "cultural barometer" to ensure Kiranmala's visual representation avoided stereotypes while celebrating her identity. It was crucial to all involved that Kiranmala appear active, possess clear agency, and display her brave, funny personality. They rejected images suggesting South Asian girls are passive, meditative, or decorative. The final cover shows Kiranmala mid-action, wearing a kurta paired with purple combat boots; the latter designed after Dr. DasGupta's own daughter's favorite shoes, which she often wore with salwar kameez [25]. This combination perfectly captures Kiranmala's identity as an immigrant daughter navigating multiple cultural worlds, fully belonging to both while being constrained by neither.

Dr. DasGupta's advocacy also extends to challenging book bans, and she is a founding member of Authors Against Book Bans. In this role, she has written for publications including *TIME*, where she argues that limiting children's access to diverse stories causes developmental harm [26, 27]. She notes that children who are read to, produce and understand language better and become better readers later in life, making censorship not just ideologically problematic but educationally damaging. Her pediatric training informs this advocacy; she understands children's development, knows the research on literacy and social-emotional growth, and can speak with authority about how representation in media affects young people's self-concept and understanding of others.

In interviews and public talks, including a TEDx presentation at Sarah Lawrence College titled "Narrative Humility: Listening as Social Justice," Dr. DasGupta weaves together her seemingly disparate careers into a coherent whole [1]. Medicine, narrative medicine scholarship, and children's writing all emerge from the same fundamental commitment to stories as healing practices and tools for justice. When practicing pediatrics, she would write prescriptions for reading, understanding that stories constitute medicine in the fullest sense. As a narrative medicine educator, she trains clinicians to honor patients' stories as essential components of care. As a children's author, she creates narratives of joy and power that help young readers imagine different, more just futures.

This integration of roles also appears in Dr. DasGupta's personal life, which she shares warmly in interviews and social media. She lives with her husband, their trilingual children, and their black Labrador retriever, Khushi, who is afraid of many things including plastic bags [1, 19]. When not writing, reading, or teaching, she watches cooking shows with her children. She speaks at conferences, both academic and literary, addressing audiences ranging from medical students to children's book professionals to general readers. She participates in panels on Asian American literature, social justice, narrative medicine, and the intersection of health and storytelling. Through all these activities, she models what it means to live at the intersection of what she calls "the stethoscope and the pen [1]."

Dr. DasGupta's family history of activism continues to inform her work. Her great-aunt Banalata DasGupta was a freedom fighter in 1930s India who drove cars, learned to fly airplanes, and was arrested by the British for hiding guns for revolutionary comrades. She died at age 21 from a preventable illness contracted in British prison. Dr. DasGupta's maternal grandfather, Sunil Kumar Das, was arrested at age 15 for participating in the 1930 Chittagong Armory Raid and spent seven harsh years in British prison, suffering beatings and contracting diseases that affected his health for life [5]. These stories of resistance, of people willing to sacrifice everything for justice and freedom, shape Dr. DasGupta's understanding of what storytelling can accomplish.

In her essay for WNDB titled "Remembering Our Radical Asian and Asian American Elders," Dr. DasGupta reflects on the price paid when we forget or erase the stories of those who came before us [5]. She notes how Asian Americans' own radical history—participation in civil rights movements, labor organizing, anti-war activism, revolutionary struggles—often gets erased in favor of model minority narratives that serve to divide communities of color and deny the reality of ongoing racism and resistance. Remembering these histories, telling these stories to young people, constitutes an act of political imagination and solidarity. Her "Force of Fire" series explicitly centers these themes, offering middle-grade readers narratives about anticolonial resistance, community organizing, and collective liberation.

As Dr. DasGupta has written, children's literature helps all young people imagine different tomorrows, tomorrows where we all can see ourselves represented and celebrated. The power of children's stories lies in their capacity to build more just futures. For readers who have always seen themselves centered in literature, this might seem abstract or overstated. But for those who grew up, as I did, as she did, rarely encountering characters who looked like us, who spoke like us, who navigated similar cultural worlds, the arrival of books like "The Serpent's Secret" "represents something profound. It says: you belong in stories of adventure and power and joy. Your culture is not exotic or *other* but simply one of many valid ways of being human.

For those of us navigating medicine while also loving literature, for those of us from minoritized communities who grew up inserting ourselves into stories that did not see us, for those of us who believe that justice and healing are intertwined and that stories matter profoundly to both, Dr. DasGupta's work offers validation, inspiration, and a roadmap. She shows us that it is possible to pursue multiple passions simultaneously, that our various identities and interests can reinforce rather than compete with one another, and that the work of creating more just, more healing futures requires both the stethoscope and the pen.

References

1. DasGupta S. Sayantani DasGupta [Official website]. n.d. http://www.sayantanidasgupta.com/.
2. BWJP. Women's history month 2023—Dr. Shamita Das Dasgupta. 2023, March 24. https://bwjp.org/womens-history-month-2023-dr-shamita-das-dasgupta/.
3. Harvard Pluralism Project. Manavi, Inc. n.d. https://hwpi.harvard.edu/pluralismarchive/manavi-inc.
4. Columbia SPS. Sayantani DasGupta, MD, MPH. n.d. https://sps.columbia.edu/person/sayantani-dasgupta-md-mph.
5. We Need Diverse Books. Remembering our radical Asian and Asian American elders. 2021, June 2. https://diversebooks.org/remembering-our-radical-asian-and-asian-american-elders/.

6. Amazon. Sayantani DasGupta [Author biography]. n.d. https://www.amazon.com/stores/author/B001HO9KUO/about?ccs_id=121a3747-7e19-4159-9dad-93894b3c9292.
7. DasGupta S. Her own medicine: a woman's journey from student to doctor. New York: Ballantine Books; 1999.
8. Amazon. Her Own Medicine: a woman's journey from student to doctor. n.d. https://www.amazon.com/Her-Own-Medicine-Journey-Student/dp/0449003094.
9. Columbia Division of General Medicine. Program in narrative medicine. n.d. https://www.genmed.columbia.edu/program-narrative-medicine.
10. Columbia News. Rita Charon's program: narrative medicine at Columbia. n.d. https://news.columbia.edu/news/narrative-medicine-teaches-doctors-how-listen-patients-stories.
11. Women in Medicine Legacy Foundation. Rita Charon, MD, PhD. n.d. https://www.wimlf.org/rita-charon-md-phd.
12. Columbia CSER. Sayantani DasGupta. n.d. https://cser.columbia.edu/cser-people/sayantani-dasgupta/.
13. DasGupta S. Narrative humility. Lancet. 2008;371(9617):980–1. https://www.thelancet.com/journals/lancet/article/PIIS0140-6736(08)60440-7/fulltext
14. Creative Nonfiction. Narrative medicine, narrative humility. n.d. https://creativenonfiction.org/writing/narrative-medicine-narrative-humility/.
15. Columbia MHE. Sayantani DasGupta, MPH, MD. n.d. https://www.mhe.cuimc.columbia.edu/narrative-medicine/bibliography/sayantani-dasgupta-mph-md.
16. International Society for the Study of Narrative. The Barbara Perkins and George Perkins Award. n.d. https://narrative.georgetown.edu/awards/perkins.php.
17. Sarah Lawrence College. Sayantani DasGupta. 2024. https://www.sarahlawrence.edu/faculty/dasgupta-sayantani.html.
18. DasGupta S. The serpent's secret (Kiranmala and the kingdom beyond, book 1). New York: Scholastic Press; 2018.
19. Penguin Random House. Sayantani DasGupta. n.d. https://www.penguinrandomhouse.com/authors/6431/sayantani-dasgupta/.
20. Barnes & Noble. Game of stars (Kiranmala and the Kingdom Beyond Series #2). n.d. https://www.barnesandnoble.com/w/game-of-stars-sayantani-dasgupta/1128563736.
21. Cotton Quilts. (2020, June 1). Sayantani DasGupta: read Asian and Pacific Islander American books. https://edicottonquilt.com/2020/06/01/sayantani-dasgupta-read-asian-and-pacific-islander-american-books/.
22. Bookshop.org. Force of fire (The fire queen #1). n.d. https://bookshop.org/p/books/force-of-fire-the-fire-queen-1-sayantani-dasgupta/.
23. Asian Author Alliance. Sayantani DasGupta. n.d. https://asianauthoralliance.com/a3directory/sayantani-dasgupta/.
24. Nixon M. Why we need more diversity in South Asian representation. We Need Diverse Books; 2020, December 3. https://www.diversebooks.org/blogposts/blog-post-title-one-a7bbn-z9gff-4r3zm-xgkxb-8clhm-7h74g-sb58b-2ctm9-87pay-y6dwz-6kffm-tm69z-hy4sl--f822y-mzwna-bp6wg-mymzm-k7asz-dsz94-9y7d4-nm5ty-z38y3-6gt96-mxlw8-kadae--wb4sg-5xjae-sfljr.
25. Zorba Books. An interview with children's author Sayantani Dasgupta. 2018, July 12. https://www.zorbabooks.com/nri-author-sayantani-dasgupta/.
26. DasGupta S. Banning books isn't just morally wrong. It's also unhealthy. TIME. 2024, October 19. https://time.com/7094430/book-banning-health-consequences/.
27. Locus Magazine. Spotlight on authors against book bans. 2025. https://locusmag.com/feature/spotlight-on-authors-against-book-bans/.

Chapter 18
Leana Wen, MD

In the early days of the COVID-19 pandemic, when life resembled the movie *Contagion*, and few of us were comfortable venturing out of our homes, verifiable, trustworthy news was a priceless commodity. Before Twitter verification could be purchased, public health officials who had secured the blue check of authenticity offered updates on vaccine research, virus variants and safety guidelines. Social media was a tool for news and communication, and #MedTwitter was the hub for public health and medicine. This was how I first encountered Dr. Leana Wen, who was, at the time, a columnist for the Washington Post. The pandemic underscored the necessity for the physician within public health as well as the fine line between patient advocacy and policymaking. Dr. Wen exemplifies the amalgamation of the advocate and legislator, while practicing as an Emergency Medicine attending.

Dr. Leana Wen was born Wen Linyan (温麟衍) on January 27, 1983, in Shanghai, China, into a family whose political dissent would ultimately reshape the trajectory of her entire life [1, 2]. Her father's involvement in opposition activities during an era of authoritarian suppression meant that the family lived under constant surveillance and threat. Young Leana spent her early childhood primarily raised by her grandparents while her parents navigated the dangers of challenging state authority. The events of June 1989 at Tiananmen Square, when she was only 6 years old, crystallized the impossibility of remaining in China. Her father's participation in dissident movements made persecution inevitable, and the family made the wrenching decision to flee, severing ties with extended family members—including the grandparents who had raised her—whom they would not see again for many years [1, 3].

On December 12, 1990, seven-year-old Wen Linyan arrived in the United States with her parents, carrying the English name Leana Sheryle Wen that would mark her new identity in a new country [1–3]. The family was granted political asylum, a recognition of the very real dangers they had fled. They settled initially in East Los Angeles and Compton, California, neighborhoods marked by poverty and the struggles of immigrant communities trying to establish footholds in America [1, 4]. The family arrived with 40 dollars to their names. The promises of asylum did not

O. M. Cox, *The Pen, The Stethoscope, and The Scalpel*,
https://doi.org/10.1007/978-3-032-19406-0_18

include economic security, and Wen's parents worked multiple jobs to survive. Her mother cleaned hotel rooms and worked as a video store clerk before eventually earning teaching credentials and becoming an elementary school teacher. Her father delivered newspapers and washed dishes before finding work as a technology manager for The Chinese Daily News in Los Angeles [1, 3].

Despite her parents' grueling work schedules, the family sometimes relied on food stamps and experienced periods of homelessness [1, 5]. Yet even in their most desperate circumstances, Wen's parents benefited from America's social safety net—Medicaid, food assistance, free public education—systems that would later inform her understanding of public health as infrastructure. Her mother, lacking health insurance, relied on Planned Parenthood for care, an experience that would resonate decades later when Wen herself would briefly lead that organization [6]. In 2003, after years of navigating immigration systems and building new lives, Wen and her family became U.S. citizens, formalizing their belonging in the country that had granted them asylum [2].

The seeds of Dr. Wen's medical career were planted in tragedy when she was 8 years old. A neighbor's child died during an asthma attack; a death that was preventable but occurred because the family, undocumented and afraid, did not call 911 for help [3, 4]. Dr. Wen herself suffered from asthma and tried desperately to help the child with her own inhaler, but it was too late [3]. This experience of witnessing how fear and systemic barriers could make the difference between life and death underscored that healthcare is not simply about medicine but about access, trust, and the social determinants that shape whether people can seek and receive care. She decided then that she wanted to become an emergency room physician, someone who would be there in moments of crisis, who could save lives that might otherwise be lost to preventable causes.

Dr. Wen's intellectual brilliance manifested early. At age 13, she enrolled in California State University, Los Angeles, through an early entrance program, pursuing a Bachelor of Science in biochemistry while her peers were still in middle school [2, 7]. She graduated summa cum laude in 2001 at age 18 [2]. Her trajectory through elite institutions continued: she attended Washington University School of Medicine in St. Louis, earning her MD in 2007 [2, 8]. As a medical student, she demonstrated leadership and advocacy, serving as National President of the American Medical Student Association, a role that positioned her at the intersection of medical education and health policy from the very beginning of her career [9, 10].

Dr. Wen's academic excellence earned her a Rhodes Scholarship to study at the University of Oxford, where she attended Merton College from 2007 to 2009 [2]. There, she completed two master's degrees, one in Economic and Social History (2007) and another in Modern Chinese Studies (2008–2009) [2, 8]. This dual focus reflected her understanding that medicine exists within broader economic, social, and historical contexts, and that addressing health requires engaging with these larger systems. Her study of Chinese history allowed her to examine her own family's experiences within frameworks of political economy, state power, and social transformation.

Following Oxford, Dr. Wen completed her residency in Emergency Medicine at Brigham and Women's Hospital and Massachusetts General Hospital in Boston, affiliated with Harvard Medical School, from 2009 to 2013 [1, 2]. She served as a Clinical Fellow at Harvard during this period, publishing research on emergency medicine systems, patient-centered care, and diagnostic approaches [2, 11]. Her early scholarly work examined topics ranging from emergency medicine workforce projections to the implementation of reflection rounds in residency programs. She also contributed to international emergency medicine development, co-authoring work on Africa's first emergency medicine training program at the University of Cape Town and Stellenbosch University [12].

It was during her residency and early practice that Dr. Wen began developing the ideas that would animate her first book. She observed patterns in how medicine was practiced; the increasing reliance on algorithmic approaches that reduced patients to checklists, the proliferation of unnecessary tests driven more by defensive medicine than diagnostic clarity, the erosion of the physician-patient relationship that should lie at the heart of good clinical care [1, 2]. Patients were being steered onto set diagnostic pathways before their stories were fully heard, categorized by chief complaints rather than understood as whole people with unique narratives. The art of diagnosis—of listening carefully, synthesizing information, generating hypotheses, and testing them thoughtfully—was being displaced by "cookbook medicine" that valued speed and standardization over personalized attention.

In 2013, Dr. Wen co-authored "When Doctors Don't Listen: How to Avoid Misdiagnoses and Unnecessary Tests," with Dr. Joshua Kosowsky, published by St. Martin's Press (Thomas Dunne Books) [13]. The book emerged from their shared frustration with how modern medicine's systems and incentives were undermining good doctoring. Their central premise was straightforward but radical: doctors are not listening to their patients, and this failure to listen leads to misdiagnoses, unnecessary testing, wasted resources, and worse patient outcomes [12]. They argued for returning to fundamentals; the partnership between physician and patient, the primacy of the clinical history and physical examination, the importance of working toward an actual diagnosis rather than simply ruling things out.

"When Doctors Don't Listen," challenged prevailing orthodoxies in medical practice [13]. At a time when evidence-based medicine and standardized clinical pathways were being celebrated as solutions to medical variation and error, Drs Wen and Kosowsky argued that these approaches, taken to extremes, created new problems. Algorithms gone wild, as they termed it, led to imprecise testing, muddled diagnoses, and patient confusion. The book offered practical guidance for patients on how to navigate medical encounters more effectively; asking better questions, insisting on working diagnoses, understanding test risks, demanding to be heard as individuals rather than processed as categories. For physicians, it was a call to reclaim diagnostic thinking, to resist the pressure to simply follow recipes, and to remember that listening and healing require engaging with the person, not just the presenting complaint.

The book garnered significant attention and praise. The New York Times called it "a superb analysis of how doctors listen and think, and offer detailed suggestions for how they could do both better [13, 14]." The Wall Street Journal noted that "Leana Wen and Joshua Kosowsky, emergency physicians at Brigham and Women's Hospital in Boston and Harvard University, urge patients to assert their voice [14]." The book became a bestseller and established Dr. Wen as an influential voice in conversations about patient-centered care and medical reform.

Following residency, Dr. Wen worked as an emergency physician at Brigham and Women's Hospital and Massachusetts General Hospital before moving to Washington, DC, to join the emergency department at George Washington University Hospital [2]. She became a professor and Director of Patient-Centered Care Research at George Washington University, continuing her clinical practice while also engaging in research, teaching, and consultation [15]. She served as a consultant to the World Health Organization, the Brookings Institution, and the China Medical Board, bringing her expertise in emergency systems and patient advocacy to international audiences [1, 12, 15].

In 2014, at age 31, Dr. Wen was approached about a position that would dramatically expand her platform and influence: Baltimore City Health Commissioner [4]. The role would lead the nation's oldest continuously operating public health department, serving a city of over 600,000 residents facing profound health challenges including one of the nation's highest rates of infant mortality, widespread lead poisoning, gun violence, HIV, and a surging opioid epidemic that was claiming hundreds of lives annually [16]. Friends and mentors encouraged her to apply despite her youth and relative lack of public health administration experience. She decided to take the chance.

Dr. Wen was appointed Baltimore City Health Commissioner on January 15, 2015, by Mayor Stephanie Rawlings-Blake [16]. She could not have anticipated that just 3 months into her tenure, the city would erupt in protests and civil unrest following the death of Freddie Gray, a 25-year-old Black man who died from injuries sustained while in police custody [16]. The uprising that followed forced the city and the nation to confront systemic racism, police violence, and the devastating effects of decades of disinvestment in Black communities [4]. Dr. Wen leveraged this moment to reframe public health's role, arguing that police brutality, poverty, lead poisoning, educational inequity, and violence were all public health issues requiring public health solutions. If we care about children's education, she argued, we must address lead poisoning in their homes. If we care about public safety, we must address mental health and addiction [1, 16].

Over nearly 4 years as Health Commissioner, Dr. Wen led Baltimore's public health department through ambitious, often controversial initiatives that garnered both national recognition and local resistance [16]. Her signature achievement was Baltimore's aggressive response to the opioid epidemic, which had reached crisis levels. In 2015, over 260 people in Baltimore City died from heroin-related overdoses. By 2017, that number had risen to 761 deaths, more than the city's homicide rate, which itself was among the nation's highest. Dr. Wen declared opioid overdose a public health emergency and implemented what became known as Baltimore's "3-Pillars" approach to combating opioid addiction [16].

The first pillar focused on saving lives immediately through expanded access to naloxone, the opioid overdose reversal medication. In one of the most aggressive naloxone distribution campaigns in the country, Dr. Wen issued a "Standing Order" that essentially made naloxone available over-the-counter to any Baltimore resident [16]. This unprecedented move allowed anyone to obtain naloxone at pharmacies without an individual prescription. The health department trained over 14,000 people in naloxone administration in the first year alone, conducting trainings in public markets, drug courts, and with police officers. This approach was controversial—critics worried it would enable drug use—but it was grounded in public health evidence that naloxone saves lives without increasing substance use [16].

The second pillar addressed improving access to addiction treatment [16]. Dr. Wen pushed for medication-assisted treatment using buprenorphine, methadone, and naltrexone, fighting against stigma that positioned these evidence-based medications as merely substituting one addiction for another. She advocated for eliminating barriers to treatment, expanding capacity, and treating addiction as the medical disease it is rather than a moral failing or criminal justice issue. This required challenging deeply entrenched attitudes, including within the medical community itself, about addiction and who deserves treatment.

The third pillar focused on education, for patients, families, communities, and prescribers. The health department launched public education campaigns including "DontDie.org" and "Bmore in Control," designed to reduce stigma and increase awareness of addiction as a treatable disease [16]. Dr. Wen sent letters to every physician in Baltimore City encouraging more judicious opioid prescribing and the co-prescribing of naloxone with opioids. She led a coalition of over 40 city health commissioners and state health directors to petition the FDA to require black box warnings when opioids and benzodiazepines are prescribed together, a combination responsible for 33% of unintentional prescription opioid overdose deaths.

Dr. Wen's work in Baltimore attracted national attention. She testified before the U.S. Senate HELP Committee and the House Oversight and Government Reform Committee, educating federal lawmakers about local-level needs and evidence-based interventions [16]. In March 2016, she was invited to the White House to join President Barack Obama and CNN's Dr. Sanjay Gupta on a panel discussion about the opioid crisis, where she spoke about Baltimore's response. Congressman Elijah Cummings, who represented Baltimore, cited Dr. Wen's efforts extensively and sought her partnership in crafting national legislation. The U.S. Surgeon General, Dr. Vivek Murthy, visited Baltimore to highlight the city's innovative approaches [16].

Beyond the opioid crisis, Dr. Wen championed treating gun violence as a public health issue, applying epidemiological methods typically used for infectious disease to patterns of violence [16]. She declared racism a public health crisis, arguing that racial discrimination creates health disparities through stress, environmental exposures, differential access to care, and intergenerational trauma. She implemented programs to reduce infant mortality, which fell to record lows during her tenure. She established a program providing glasses to all Baltimore City school children who needed them, recognizing that vision problems affect learning and that many families could not afford corrective lenses. She convened the Baltimore Statement on the Importance of Childhood Vaccinations in response to anti-vaccine movements. She successfully advocated to ban the sale of powdered alcohol in Maryland and synthetic drugs in Baltimore.

These accomplishments came at significant personal and professional cost. Dr. Wen navigated political pressures, budget constraints, and resistance from those who disagreed with public health approaches to issues traditionally handled through criminal justice or moral frameworks. She faced criticism from multiple directions, from those who thought her approaches too progressive and from those who wanted more radical change. Her memoir "Lifelines," describes the compromises required, the frustrations of bureaucracy, and the toll of fighting for evidence-based policies in politicized environments [17].

In September 2018, Dr. Wen announced she would leave Baltimore to become the sixth president and CEO of Planned Parenthood, one of the nation's largest reproductive health care providers [6]. She stepped down as Health Commissioner on October 12, 2018, having served nearly 4 years. Her tenure in Baltimore had saved an estimated 3000 lives from opioid overdose according to health department modeling, reduced infant mortality to record lows, and established Baltimore as a national leader in innovative public health approaches. She expressed pride in her team's accomplishments while acknowledging that leaving a job she loved carried costs.

Dr. Wen's time at Planned Parenthood would prove brief and contentious. She assumed leadership at a precarious moment: the Trump administration had implemented policies restricting access to family planning services, conservative activists were pushing increasingly aggressive restrictions on abortion access, and Planned Parenthood was facing existential political and legal challenges [18]. Dr. Wen envisioned expanding Planned Parenthood's health services beyond reproductive care, emphasizing its role in providing primary care, STI testing and treatment, cancer screenings, and other services to underserved communities. She wanted to position the organization as a comprehensive healthcare provider rather than primarily an abortion rights advocacy organization [1, 18].

This vision put her at odds with Planned Parenthood's board of directors and many of its core supporters. In the midst of escalating attacks on abortion rights, they wanted a leader focused on political advocacy and defense of abortion access specifically [18]. The philosophical differences proved irreconcilable. In July 2019, just 8 months after beginning her tenure, Dr. Wen was removed as president by the board in what she described as a secret meeting. In a statement, she expressed her belief that the organization's future depended on doubling down on abortion rights advocacy while she had wanted to emphasize the broader healthcare mission. The departure was painful and public, generating significant media attention and debate about Planned Parenthood's strategic direction.

The timing proved fortuitous in one respect: as Dr. Wen was navigating her departure from Planned Parenthood in mid-2019, she could not have known that within months, the world would face a pandemic that would make public health expertise more visible and more contested than at any time in modern history. When

COVID-19 emerged in late 2019 and began spreading globally in early 2020, Dr. Wen was positioned to step into a critical role as a public health communicator and analyst.

In early 2020, Dr. Wen joined George Washington University as a visiting professor of health policy and management at the Milken Institute School of Public Health, where she also became a distinguished fellow at the Fitzhugh Mullan Institute for Health Workforce Equity [15]. She began writing regularly for The Washington Post, first as a contributing op-ed writer in 2019, then formalizing her role as a columnist in 2020 when she launched "The Checkup with Dr. Wen," a twice-weekly newsletter on public health and healthcare [19]. She also became a medical analyst for CNN, appearing frequently on air to discuss COVID-19 and other public health topics [20].

Throughout the pandemic, Dr. Wen emerged as one of the most visible physician voices in mainstream media, appearing on CNN, NPR, PBS, BBC, and MSNBC, and writing extensively for The Washington Post [21]. She was asked to testify four times to Congress during the COVID-19 pandemic, including twice to the Select Subcommittee on the Coronavirus Crisis [8]. Her commentary spanned the full range of pandemic issues: vaccine development and distribution, masking policies, school closures, travel restrictions, risk stratification, the balance between public health measures and economic/social costs, mental health impacts, and the politics of pandemic response.

Dr. Wen's pandemic commentary generated both appreciation and controversy. She consistently emphasized evidence-based approaches, risk assessment, and practical guidance for individuals navigating uncertain circumstances. As someone who had participated in a Johnson & Johnson vaccine clinical trial (receiving either vaccine or placebo, never learning which), she spoke from personal experience about vaccine development. Her family's own bout with COVID-19—where she cared for her husband and children while fortuitously not contracting the virus herself—informed her understanding of household transmission dynamics [22].

However, Dr. Wen also drew criticism from some public health advocates for positions they viewed as insufficiently cautious or excessively focused on individual risk rather than community protection. Her emphasis on targeted interventions based on risk stratification, her calls to reassess certain restrictions as vaccines became available, and her arguments about the costs of prolonged school closures put her at odds with those advocating more stringent measures [1, 22]. In 2023, she received significant attention for a piece arguing that COVID deaths were being overcounted, a position that some critics viewed as validation of earlier claims they had dismissed as conspiracy theories, while others defended her nuanced argument about the distinction between dying "from" COVID versus dying "with" COVID [23].

This willingness to take positions that challenged both conservative and progressive orthodoxies has characterized Dr. Wen's public presence. She has argued against excessive testing when evidence doesn't support it, while also calling for more widespread testing when outbreaks demand it. She has supported vaccine mandates while also emphasizing informed consent and addressing vaccine hesitancy through education rather than coercion. She has called out failures of the Trump administration's pandemic response while also criticizing aspects of Biden administration policies. In March 2025, she wrote an op-ed supporting Trump's nominees for NIH and FDA leadership, Jay Bhattacharya and Marty Makary, based on their qualifications and her assessment of needed reforms, despite significant criticism from colleagues who opposed these nominations [24].

This independent stance reflects Dr. Wen's stated philosophy, expressed in "Lifelines" : "I have little tolerance for those who value purity over practical action [17]." She positions herself as a pragmatist focused on achieving concrete improvements in health outcomes rather than maintaining ideological consistency. Whether this approach represents admirable independence or troubling inconsistency remains debated, but it has undeniably made her a prominent and influential voice in public health discourse.

Her memoire, "Lifelines: A Doctor's Journey in the Fight for Public Health," was published in 2021, with Metropolitan Books [17]. The book interweaves her personal story—from political asylum seeker to Rhodes Scholar to Baltimore Health Commissioner to pandemic commentator—with her vision for public health's crucial role in addressing not just disease but poverty, racism, violence, and inequality. She articulates the principle that guides her work: "Public health saved your life today, you just don't know it." Good public health is invisible; it becomes visible only in its absence, when systems fail or are underfunded. The pandemic, she argues, laid bare the consequences of decades of public health neglect.

"Lifelines" received strong reviews. Kirkus called it "a moving account of an impressively fruitful life" and "a provocative exploration of public health from an immigrant physician and expert's point of view [5]." Dr. Sanjay Gupta wrote that it is Dr. Wen's "origin story" as a "public health superhero, destined to make profound changes in our world [25]." Senator Barbara Mikulski praised it for giving readers "a crash course in the nuts and bolts of policy and politics" while making them "into a believer in the power of public health [25]." The book captured both Dr. Wen's remarkable trajectory and her passionate advocacy for viewing health through structural lenses that address social determinants.

The book also reveals personal dimensions of Wen's life and challenges that might not be apparent from her polished media appearances. She describes overcoming a stutter through intensive therapy, work that helped her develop the precise enunciation and careful speech patterns that characterize her communication style. This disclosure surprised many who had watched her speak fluently on television, illustrating how invisible disability can be and how much effort goes into performances of competence that others experience as effortless.

Dr. Wen's family life centers on her husband, Sebastian Neil Walker, a South African native whom she married in 2012 (with a blessing ceremony in Cape Town and later a legal ceremony in Boston) [26]. Walker is an Emmy Award-winning journalist who has worked as a correspondent and Middle East bureau chief for VICE News Tonight on HBO. They have two children: a son named Eli born in 2017 and a daughter named Isabelle born in 2020 [6, 20]. Balancing parenting, clinical medicine, academic work, writing, media appearances, and advocacy requires extraordinary time management and support systems. Dr. Wen has spoken about the challenges of being a working mother in demanding fields, the guilt of time away from children, and the ways motherhood has deepened her commitment to healthcare access and family-friendly policies.

Dr. Wen maintains her emergency medicine board certification and describes herself as a practicing physician, though her clinical work has necessarily been limited by her other commitments [1, 20]. She serves as a nonresident senior fellow at the Brookings Institution, where she contributes to policy research and recommendations. She has served on numerous advisory boards for governmental, non-profit, academic, and corporate entities including the Patient-Centered Outcomes Research Institute, Council on Graduate Medical Education, Lown Institute, and Accolade Inc. [12]

Her honors and recognitions are extensive. She has been named one of TIME magazine's 100 Most Influential People (2019) [27], Modern Healthcare's 50 Most Influential Physician Executives (multiple years), and Modern Healthcare's Top 25 Minority Physician Executives (2017–2018) [1]. She received Governing magazine's Public Officials of the Year award (2017), the World Economic Forum's Young Global Leaders designation, and the American Public Health Association's highest award for local public health work [12]. She is a Fellow of the American Academy of Emergency Medicine and the Academy of Medicine. She has received honorary doctorates and delivered commencement addresses at numerous institutions including the University of Maryland School of Medicine, Johns Hopkins Bloomberg School of Public Health, and Washington University School of Medicine [12].

As a writer, Dr. Wen has authored dozens of articles in scientific publications including The Lancet, JAMA, Health Affairs, British Medical Journal, Academic Emergency Medicine, and Western Journal of Emergency Medicine [12, 15, 20]. Her work spans clinical emergency medicine, public health policy, addiction medicine, health equity, and pandemic response. She has given six TEDx and TEDMED talks, including presentations on public health as an urban solution, physician transparency, and the opioid crisis [28].

Dr. Wen's impact on medicine operates through multiple channels. As Health Commissioner of Baltimore, she demonstrated that aggressive public health interventions like widespread naloxone distribution can save thousands of lives [16]. Her emphasis on treating addiction as a disease rather than a crime, on racism and violence as public health issues, and on addressing social determinants rather than just individual behaviors has influenced how public health departments approach these challenges. Many jurisdictions have adopted variations of Baltimore's naloxone standing order and 3-pillar approach to the opioid epidemic.

Through "When Doctors Don't Listen," Dr. Wen influenced conversations about patient-centered care, diagnostic reasoning, and the problems with algorithmic medicine. The book empowered patients to advocate for themselves more effectively while challenging physicians to reclaim the art of medicine. Through "Lifelines," she provided both a memoir of immigrant achievement and a manifesto for public health's essential role in creating just, healthy communities. Through her

Washington Post column and CNN appearances, she has reached millions of people with evidence-based public health guidance, making complex health policy accessible and relevant to daily decision-making.

For medical trainees and early-career physicians considering how to use their training to maximum effect, Dr. Wen offers a model of versatility and ambition. She demonstrates that physicians can move between clinical practice, academic work, public service, writing, and advocacy without abandoning medicine. The common thread connecting these seemingly disparate activities is the fundamental commitment to reducing suffering and promoting health; whether through treating individual patients, implementing population-level interventions, shaping policy, or educating the public.

Dr. Wen's story also illustrates the ongoing importance of immigrant contributions to American medicine and public health. From fleeing political persecution in China to becoming one of the nation's most influential public health voices, her trajectory embodies possibilities that immigration enables. Her lived experience of poverty, reliance on social safety nets, and navigating healthcare as an uninsured patient informs her advocacy in ways that cannot be replicated through academic study alone. The diversity of perspective and experience she brings, as an immigrant, as a woman, as someone who has experienced both poverty and professional success, enriches public health discourse and policy development.

Dr. Leana Wen exemplifies the physician-writer-advocate who refuses to accept that medicine is only about individual patient encounters, that writing is only about personal expression, or that advocacy is someone else's responsibility. She demonstrates that physicians can and should engage with the full spectrum of factors affecting health, from the molecular to the societal. Her career challenges medical trainees to think expansively about what physician work can encompass and how medical training can serve broader purposes than individual clinical practice.

References

1. Wen L. Lifelines: a doctor's journey in the fight for public health [Official website]. n.d. https://drleanawen.com/.
2. Merton College, Oxford. Dr Leana Wen, MD (2007). 2021. https://www.carnegie.org/awards/honoree/leana-wen/.
3. Carnegie Corporation of New York. Leana Wen | 2019 Great Immigrants. 2019. https://www.carnegie.org/awards/honoree/leana-wen/.
4. Governing Magazine. Public officials of the year: Leana Wen. 2017. https://www.governing.com/poy/gov-leana-wen.html.
5. Kirkus Reviews. Lifelines [Book review]. 2021, June. https://www.kirkusreviews.com/book-reviews/leana-wen/lifelines-wen/.
6. Planned Parenthood Federation of America. Planned Parenthood announcement. 2018, September 12 https://www.plannedparenthood.org/about-us/newsroom/press-releases/planned-parenthood-announcement.
7. California State University, Los Angeles. Cal State LA alumna to head Planned Parenthood. 2018 https://www.calstatela.edu/univ/ppa/publicat/cal-state-la-alumna-head-planned-parenthood.

8. George Washington University Milken Institute School of Public Health. Leana Wen joins Milken Institute School of Public Health. 2019, August. https://publichealth.gwu.edu/leana-wen-joins-milken-institute-school-public-health.
9. Washington University in St. Louis, The Source. Medical students elected to national positions in AMSA. 2005, March. https://source.washu.edu/2005/03/medical-students-elected-to-national-positions-in-amsa/.
10. American Medical Student Association (AMSA). Past AMSA presidents. 2024. https://www.amsa.org/about/history/past-amsa-presidents/.
11. Bipartisan Policy Center. Dr. Leana Wen. 2024. https://bipartisanpolicy.org/person/leana-wen/.
12. Wen LS. Leana S. Wen, M.D. M.Sc. FAAEM [Curriculum vitae]. Brookings Institution; 2023, September. https://www.brookings.edu/wp-content/uploads/2024/01/Dr-Leana-Wen-Academic-CV-September-2023.pdf.
13. Wen L, Kosowsky JM. When doctors don't listen: how to avoid misdiagnoses and unnecessary tests. New York: St. Martin's Press; 2013.
14. Wen LS, Kosowsky JM. When doctors don't listen: how to avoid misdiagnoses and unnecessary tests. Thomas Dunne Books/St. Martin's Griffin; 2014. https://www.amazon.com/When-Doctors-Dont-Listen-Misdiagnoses/dp/1250048486.
15. Mullan Institute, George Washington University. Leana Wen [Faculty page]. 2024. https://faculty.smhs.gwu.edu/leana-sheryle-wen.
16. Baltimore City Health Department. Press releases and public statements. 2015–2018.
17. Wen L. Lifelines: a doctor's journey in the fight for public health. New York: Metropolitan Books/Henry Holt and Company; 2021.
18. NPR. Planned Parenthood removes Leana Wen as president after less than a year. 2019, July 16. https://www.npr.org/2019/07/16/742390932/planned-parenthood-removes-leana-wen-as-president-after-less-than-a-year.
19. The Washington Post. The Checkup with Dr. Wen [Newsletter]. 2020–present. https://www.washingtonpost.com/newsletters/the-checkup-with-dr-wen/.
20. Brookings Institution. Dr. Leana Wen. 2024, January 31. https://www.brookings.edu/people/dr leana wen/.
21. World Economic Forum. Leana Wen. 2024. https://www.weforum.org/people/leana-wen/.
22. Wen L. [@DrLeanaWen]. Tweets [X profile]. X. n.d. https://x.com/DrLeanaWen.
23. Goedert S. Professor receives backlash for commentary bashing US pandemic response. The GW Hatchet. 2023, February 13. https://gwhatchet.com/2023/02/13/professor-receives-backlash-for-commentary-bashing-us-pandemic-response/.
24. Wen LS. The NIH and FDA nominees are surprisingly strong. The Washington Post. 2025, March 11. https://www.washingtonpost.com/opinions/2025/03/11/bhattacharya-makary-nih-fda-trump/.
25. Wen L. Lifelines: a doctor's journey in the fight for public health. Metropolitan Books/Henry Holt and Company; 2021. https://www.amazon.com/Lifelines-Doctors-Journey-Public-Health/dp/1250186234.
26. Mallozz, VM. Leana Wen, Sebastian Walker—weddings. The New York Times. 2012, February 12. https://www.nytimes.com/2012/02/12/fashion/weddings/leana-wen-sebastian-walker-weddings.html.
27. TIME. Leana Wen: The 100 most influential people of 2019. 2019, April. https://time.com/collection/100-most-influential-people-2019/5567751/leana-wen/.
28. TED. Leana Wen [Speaker profile]. n.d. https://www.ted.com/speakers/leana_wen

Chapter 19
Elizabeth Blackwell, MD

Part of my upbringing involved the concept of "Holiday Work," which was not assigned by the school in any capacity, but was secondary to my parent's belief that we only need approximately 2 weeks of "vacation," after which we should be "exercising our minds." And so, although my childhood memories of vacation included the beach house in Diani, Kenya, or seeing elephants in the London Zoo, they also involved solving mathematical proofs in hotel rooms and writing essays about important figures in the Forest Hill Library. This was my first introduction to Dr. Elizabeth Blackwell. At the time, I likely selected her because she shared my mother's English name and after I was done reading, I was prepared to forge a path into the world of medicine. Geneva Medical College, where she earned her medical degree, was the predecessor to my medical school, and I am thrilled to rediscover her career's work after so long.

Dr. Elizabeth Blackwell was born in Bristol, England, on February 3, 1821, the third of nine children in a family that would become synonymous with progressive social reform [1–4]. Her father, Samuel Blackwell, was a sugar refiner and ardent Quaker whose beliefs in equality and education shaped the trajectory of his children's lives [5]. Unlike most families of the era, the Blackwell children received equal education regardless of gender, taught by private tutors in subjects ranging from mathematics to literature [4]. This early exposure to intellectual parity planted the seeds for Dr. Blackwell's revolutionary pursuit.

The Blackwell family immigrated to the United States in 1832 when Elizabeth was 11, settling first in New York before moving to Cincinnati, Ohio [2, 5]. Samuel Blackwell died shortly after the family's arrival in Ohio in 1838, leaving the family penniless during a national financial crisis [2–5]. The eldest Blackwell children, including Elizabeth, took up the predominantly female profession of teaching to support the family [5]. Teaching, while respectable, was one of the few "appropriate" careers for women, and yet Elizabeth found it profoundly unsuitable to her temperament and ambitions. The catalyst for Elizabeth's medical career came from an unexpected source. A close friend who was dying suggested that her suffering

O. M. Cox, *The Pen, The Stethoscope, and The Scalpel*,
https://doi.org/10.1007/978-3-032-19406-0_19

would have been lessened had her physician been a woman. This moment of vulnerability, and recognition of the profound discomfort experienced by women under the care of male physicians in an era of extreme modesty, ignited something in Elizabeth [5, 6].

Initially, Elizabeth herself found the prospect distasteful. She later wrote that she "hated everything connected with the body, and could not bear the sight of a medical book… the very thought of dwelling on the physical structure of the body and its various ailments filled me with disgust [5, 6]." How many of us in medicine can relate to this initial recoil? The body, with all its vulnerabilities and indignities, is not always an easy subject of study. Yet Elizabeth persevered, driven by what she described as a "great moral struggle;" the attraction to a fight that needed fighting.

The barriers she faced were monumental. She applied to numerous prominent medical schools but was rejected by all of them initially [5]. Medical education in the 1840s was largely an apprenticeship system, and while some women did practice medicine unlicensed, no accredited institution would formally admit a woman. Elizabeth sought mentorship from physician friends and studied privately, but the door to legitimate medical education remained closed.

Enter Geneva Medical College in Upstate New York. The faculty, wishing to avoid the politically charged decision, put her application to a student vote, stating that if even one student voted no, she would be barred from admission [2, 5, 7]. They were certain the all-male student body would reject her. Instead, the medical students voted unanimously to admit her, viewing it as a joke, never expecting a woman to actually attend or complete the rigorous course of study [7].

Walking those halls as a first-year medical student myself, I thought often of Elizabeth Blackwell. Geneva Medical College would eventually become part of SUNY Upstate Medical University, and the building where she studied still stands [7]. I imagined her entering those same lecture halls, facing not just the challenge of mastering anatomy, pharmacology, and pathology, but doing so while being treated as a spectacle, an anomaly, perhaps a joke. Professors forced her to sit separately at lectures and often excluded her from labs; local townspeople shunned her as a "bad" woman for defying her gender role.

Yet Dr. Blackwell excelled. Through intellectual rigor and unwavering determination, she graduated first in her class on January 23, 1849, becoming the first woman in America to graduate from medical school [2, 5, 7]. Her education was far from complete, however, and Dr. Blackwell traveled to Europe to continue her training, seeking positions in the prestigious hospitals of Paris and London. While a resident at La Maternité in Paris, she contracted purulent ophthalmia from an infant patient, an infection that cost her 6 months of illness and the sight of one eye [4, 5, 7, 8]. The eye was eventually surgically removed, ending her ambitions for a career in surgery [5, 7, 8]. Here was another door closed by circumstance, another dream deferred. But Dr. Blackwell adapted, as physicians must, redirecting her path while maintaining her mission.

In 1858, largely through the influence of Sir James Paget, she became the first woman entered on the British Medical Register, making her not only America's first female doctor but Britain's as well [3–5]. This dual distinction speaks to her transatlantic influence and the universality of the barriers women faced in medicine.

Returning to New York in 1851, Dr. Blackwell found that discrimination against female physicians meant few patients and difficulty practicing in hospitals and clinics. She opened a small dispensary near Tompkins Square to treat poor women, demonstrating early on her commitment to underserved populations [9]. In 1857, she expanded this work by founding the New York Infirmary for Women and Children with her younger sister Dr. Emily Blackwell, who had also earned a medical degree. By 1866, this institution was treating nearly 7000 patients annually [9–11].

The establishment of the Women's Medical College of the New York Infirmary in 1868 represented another milestone [2]. It incorporated Dr. Blackwell's innovative ideas about medical education; a four-year training period with much more extensive clinical training than previously required. This was revolutionary pedagogy, emphasizing practical, hands-on experience over rote memorization [2]. As someone who learned medicine in an era that prizes clinical exposure, I recognize that Dr. Blackwell was advocating for what we now consider best practices over 150 years ago.

In 1869, Dr. Blackwell returned permanently to England, leaving her sister Emily in charge of the American institutions [1–3]. She became a professor of gynecology at the London School of Medicine for Women in 1875, which she had helped establish alongside Florence Nightingale, Sophia Jex-Blake, and Elizabeth Garrett Anderson [1–5]. Her influence extended beyond individual patient care to the systemic transformation of medical education and institutional access for women.

Dr. Blackwell was also a prolific author, producing at least 10 major books and numerous pamphlets throughout her career [2]. In 1852, she published "The Laws of Life with Special Reference to the Physical Education of Girls," a volume examining the physical and mental development of young women. This was followed by "Medicine as a Profession for Women in 1860" and "Address on the Medical Education of Women in 1864," works that directly advocated for women's entry into the medical profession [12–17].

Her most important book was "Counsel to Parents on the Moral Education of Children," published in 1876, which was translated into French and German [2]. She also wrote "The Laws of Life" (1852), "The Religion of Health" (1869), "Wrong and Right Methods of Dealing with Social Evil" (1883), "The Human Element in Sex" (1884), and "Essays in Medical Sociology" (1902). Her writings ranged from practical medical advice to moral philosophy, from public health advocacy to education reform. But it is her autobiography, "Pioneer Work in Opening the Medical Profession to Women," published in 1895, that stands as her most famous and enduring literary contribution [12–17]. She writes not merely to document her own achievements but to illuminate the path for those who would follow [11].

Throughout her later years, Dr. Blackwell was an active participant in many reform movements including moral reform, sexuality, hygiene, medical education, preventative medicine, women's suffrage, government morals, and the abolition of slavery [1–5]. She was particularly passionate about preventative medicine and public health, recognizing that proper hygiene and sanitation could prevent more illness than treatment could cure. During the Civil War, she helped establish the US Sanitary Commission, applying these principles to military healthcare [18].

In 1907, Dr. Blackwell fell while on vacation in Scotland and suffered a head injury that permanently impaired her mental faculties [4]. It is a cruel irony that a mind so sharp, so revolutionary, should be dimmed by such an accident. She died at her home in Hastings, England on May 31, 1910, at the age of 89, after suffering a stroke [4], and was buried in the churchyard of St Munn's Parish Church at Kilmun on Holy Loch in the west of Scotland [4]. By 1910, women accounted for approximately 6% of U.S. physicians, with an estimated 9015 female physicians practicing in America [19].

Dr. Elizabeth Blackwell's impact on medicine is immeasurable. She didn't merely open a door that had been closed to women; she kicked it down, walked through, and then held it open for thousands of others. She demonstrated that women possessed the intellectual capacity, physical stamina, and emotional fortitude to excel in medicine. She established institutions that trained generations of female physicians. She advocated for educational reforms that improved medical training for everyone. She championed public health and preventative care decades before these became mainstream priorities.

Her literary legacy is equally significant. Through her extensive writings, Dr. Blackwell created a body of work that served multiple purposes: documenting the struggles women faced in entering medicine, providing practical guidance for aspiring female physicians, advocating for educational and social reforms, and articulating a philosophy of medicine that emphasized prevention, hygiene, and holistic care. Her autobiography remains an essential primary source for understanding both nineteenth-century medicine and women's history.

In popular culture, Dr. Elizabeth Blackwell has been commemorated in numerous ways. She was honored with a commemorative postage stamp and Hobart and William Smith Colleges erected a statue on their campus. In 1957, "The Blackwell Story" was broadcast as part of the CBS television series Playhouse 90, with Joanne Dru playing Dr. Blackwell. More recently, a 2014 animated film, "Who Says Women Can't Be Doctors?: The Story of Elizabeth Blackwell," directed by Melissa Ellard, introduced her story to younger audiences [20]. In 2021, Janice P. Nimura published "The Doctors Blackwell," chronicling the life stories of Elizabeth and her sister Emily [20, 21–24]. And in 2025, Upstate Medical University erected a statue in her honor at the entrance to the main academic building, along with another prominent alumnae, Dr. Sarah Loguen Fraser [25].

Dr. Elizabeth Blackwell's contributions are celebrated through the Elizabeth Blackwell Medal, awarded annually to a woman who has made a significant contribution to the promotion of women in medicine [11]. In May 2018, a commemorative plaque was unveiled at the former location of the New York Infirmary for Indigent Women and Children, ensuring that her physical legacy is remembered.

Poet Jessy Randall's 2022 collection of poems about women scientists, Mathematics for Ladies, was originally inspired by her interest in Blackwell, demonstrating how Dr. Blackwell's story continues to inspire artistic creation [8].

In her writings, Dr. Blackwell frequently emphasized the interconnection between physical health and moral education, between individual wellness and social reform. She understood that medicine exists within a social context, that physicians must address not only disease but the conditions that produce disease. She advocated for hygiene education, improved living conditions for the poor, and for rational approaches to sexuality and reproduction. She was, in the truest sense, a social physician; someone who recognized that healing requires addressing both individual pathology and social determinants of health.

Reading her work now, it is evident how contemporary many of her concerns remain. We still debate the proper training of physicians, the balance between clinical experience and theoretical knowledge. We still grapple with issues of access to healthcare, particularly for marginalized populations. We still confront barriers to entry in medicine based on gender, race, socioeconomic status, and other factors. Dr. Blackwell's voice, speaking across more than a century, remains remarkably relevant.

Her story also serves as a reminder of the power of mentorship and mutual support. Dr. Blackwell did not succeed alone. She had the support of her family, particularly her sisters Anna, Marian, and Emily. She was mentored by physicians who recognized her potential despite prevailing prejudices. She, in turn, became a mentor to others, including Elizabeth Garrett Anderson and Marie Zakrzewska [3]. This chain of support, this commitment to lifting others as we climb, is essential to lasting change.

As physician-writers, we inherit Dr. Elizabeth Blackwell's legacy in multiple ways. We inherit the opportunity to practice medicine that she fought to secure. We inherit the responsibility to document our experiences, to advocate for change, to use our words alongside our stethoscopes. We inherit the understanding that medicine is both art and science, that healing requires empathy alongside evidence, that our stories matter.

Today, women comprise more than half of medical school matriculants in the United States [19]. We have female department chairs, deans, surgeons general. The question is no longer whether women can be doctors but how medicine can better support all of its practitioners, regardless of gender. These are good problems to have—problems of refinement rather than revolution—but we face them only because Dr. Elizabeth Blackwell and women like her refused to accept the limitations imposed on them. Dr. Elizabeth Blackwell reminds us that medicine is not just about treating disease but about healing society, that writing is not just about recording events but about shaping futures, and that a single life, lived with purpose and courage, can alter the trajectory of history itself.

References

1. National Library of Medicine. Biography: Dr. Elizabeth Blackwell. n.d. https://www.nlm.nih.gov/exhibition/changing-the-face-of-medicine/physicians/biography_elizabeth_blackwell.html.
2. Britannica. Elizabeth Blackwell. Encyclopedia Britannica. n.d. https://www.britannica.com/biography/Elizabeth-Blackwell.
3. Oxford Dictionary of National Biography. Blackwell, Elizabeth (1821–1910), physician. n.d. https://www.oxforddnb.com/display/10.1093/ref:odnb/9780198614128.001.0001/odnb-9780198614128-e-31912.
4. Encyclopedia.com. Elizabeth Blackwell (1821–1910) biography. n.d. https://www.encyclopedia.com/people/medicine/medicine-biographies/elizabeth-blackwell.
5. Hobart and William Smith Colleges. Elizabeth Blackwell biography. n.d. https://www.hws.edu/about/history/elizabeth-blackwell/biography.aspx.
6. HISTORY. Elizabeth Blackwell becomes first woman to receive medical degree. n.d. https://www.history.com/this-day-in-history/elizabeth-blackwell-becomes-first-woman-to-receive-medical-degree.
7. SUNY Upstate Medical University. Women in medicine and science at Upstate: Elizabeth Blackwell MD. n.d. https://guides.upstate.edu/women-in-medicine/elizabeth-blackwell.
8. Hobart and William Smith Colleges. Celebrating 150 years of women in medicine. n.d. https://www.hws.edu/about/history/elizabeth-blackwell/150-years.aspx.
9. National Library of Medicine. Changing the face of medicine: Biography of Elizabeth Blackwell. n.d. https://cfmedicine.nlm.nih.gov/physicians/biography_35.html.
10. NewYork-Presbyterian. It happened here: Dr. Elizabeth Blackwell. n.d. https://healthmatters.nyp.org/happened-dr-elizabeth-blackwell/.
11. Life in the Fast Lane. Elizabeth Blackwell. Medical Eponym Library; 2024, September 5. https://litfl.com/elizabeth-blackwell/.
12. Blackwell E. The laws of life, with special reference to the physical education of girls. George P. Putnam. 1852. https://archive.org/details/61360800R.nlm.nih.gov.
13. Blackwell E. Medicine as a profession for women. Trustees of the New York Infirmary for Women; 1860. https://archive.org/details/62630060R.nlm.nih.gov.
14. Blackwell E. Counsel to parents on the moral education of their children. Hatchards; 1879. https://archive.org/details/b22354347.
15. Blackwell E. Pioneer work in opening the medical profession to women. Longmans, Green, and Co.; 1895. https://www.gutenberg.org/ebooks/65496.
16. Blackwell E. Essays in medical sociology. Ernest Bell; 1902. https://archive.org/details/39002006316815.med.yale.edu.
17. Barnes & Noble. Essays in medical sociology, volume 1 of 2. n.d. https://www.barnesandnoble.com/w/essays-in-medical-sociology-volume-1-of-2-elizabeth-blackwell/1143237661.
18. Essential Civil War Curriculum. The US Sanitary Commission. n.d. https://www.essentialcivilwarcurriculum.com/the-us-sanitary-commission.html.
19. Nallamotu S, Vankayalapati A, Paruchuri S. Dr. Elizabeth Blackwell (1821–1910): opening doors to women in medicine. Cureus. 2024;16(10):e71899. https://pmc.ncbi.nlm.nih.gov/articles/PMC11574509/.
20. IMDb. Who says women can't be doctors?: The story of Elizabeth Blackwell. 2014. https://www.imdb.com/title/tt9728294/.
21. Nimura JP. The doctors Blackwell [Author website]. n.d. https://www.janicenimura.com/doctors-blackwell/.
22. Nimura JP. The doctors Blackwell: how two pioneering sisters brought medicine to women and women to medicine. W.W. Norton & Company; 2021. https://wwnorton.com/books/9780393635546.

23. Amazon. The doctors Blackwell: How two pioneering sisters brought medicine to women and women to medicine. n.d. https://www.amazon.com/Doctors-Blackwell-Pioneering-Sisters-Medicine/dp/0393635546.
24. Kirkus Reviews. The doctors Blackwell [Review]. n.d. https://www.kirkusreviews.com/book-reviews/janice-p-nimura/the-doctors-blackwell/.
25. Albanese J. Upstate honors pioneering women with life-sized bronze statues welcoming students to campus. SUNY Upstate News. 2025, October 23. https://www.upstate.edu/news/articles/2025/2025-10-23-blackwell-fraser-statues.php.

Chapter 20
Michele Harper, MD

An interesting development in medical training has been the growth of students who are so-called, "non-traditional. " This group, however, is typically quite traditional for the world outside of medicine. They are former bankers, teachers, mechanics, and even parents. They have crossed milestones from their first child to their first home, bankruptcy, divorce, and marriage. This conglomerate of various life-stages offers the unique opportunity to be eyewitness to many of life's lessons outside of medical training. Some of my friends had entered the hallowed halls of Middle Age before our clinical rotations and brought with them invaluable lived experience to their patient care. Others arrived with the multitasking acumen that comes from raising children. And so, it is certainly true that those of us who have spent time experiencing adulthood prior to medical school, are non-traditional compared to those of us who walked a continuous path from undergraduate studies. However, there is significant benefit to having physicians who have navigated the rocky shores of life in the same way as many of their patients. Not simply for the sake of camaraderie, but because they personally understand the driving emotions that exist in the storms, that life allots us. Dr. Michele Harper is one such doctor, who describes the journey of her healing post-divorce through her meetings with patients. Her deep empathy swells through the lines of her vivid words; "The Beauty in Breaking" is a healing journey, a painful journey, a needed journey and a reminder that sharing our journeys makes us better doctors.

Dr. Michele Harper was born in Washington, DC, and grew up within a family afflicted with abuse [1, 2]. The specifics of her childhood home life would shape not only her personal journey but also her approach to medicine in profound ways. Dr. Harper recalled one of numerous descents into darkness when her teenaged brother was fighting her father to protect her mother, a scene of violence that ultimately led to her first encounter with emergency medicine. When Michele Harper was in her teens, she got her first taste of the emergency room: "I marveled at the place, one of bright lights and dark hallways, a place so quiet and yet so throbbing with life [3]."

O. M. Cox, *The Pen, The Stethoscope, and The Scalpel*,
https://doi.org/10.1007/978-3-032-19406-0_20

Unlike some who discover medicine through illness or curiosity, Michele's path was forged in trauma. She wasn't there for an innocent childhood fall, but because her father had physically abused her brother, again [2]. In this origin story, of Dr. Harper, the emergency department became for her what it has become for so many: a place of refuge, a space where chaos could be managed, where broken things could be mended.

Yet it was that visit to the emergency room that crystalized her desire to heal and pursue medicine. "If my brother's body could be patched up, then certainly, in its own time, his spirit could mend, too." This belief in healing, both physical and spiritual, would become the cornerstone of her medical philosophy. Harper left the ED marveling, not least because of the sense of commonality she'd felt with the other people in the waiting room. "All of us had converged…to reveal our wounds, to offer up our hurt and [for] our pain to be eased," she would later observe in her memoir [2, 3].

Dr. Harper's academic path took her from the difficult circumstances of her home life to Harvard University, where she met her husband [2, 3]. Following her graduation from Harvard, she went on to earn her medical degree from the now-named Renaissance School of Medicine at Stony Brook University. Dr. Harper excelled in medical school, deciding to pursue emergency room medicine as her specialty, due largely to the immediacy of fixing broken bodies. "Unlike in the war zone that was my childhood, I would be in control of that space, providing relief or at least a reprieve to those who called out for help," she noted [2].

She is a proud graduate of the Lincoln Medical & Mental Health Center emergency medicine residency program in the South Bronx, where she received the Joel Gernsheimer Award for excellence in emergency medicine [1, 4, 5]. Lincoln Hospital in the South Bronx was not an easy training ground. It is one of those places where you see everything, where the full spectrum of human suffering and resilience plays out shift after shift. She completed the demanding training program, and was on the cusp of professional and personal satisfaction, with her then husband. But life, as it does, had other breaks planned for Dr. Harper. Although they had stayed together through the rigors of medical school and the vagaries of residency, just two months prior to her beginning her commitment as an attending in central Philadelphia, her husband admitted that he would not be moving with her. Her marriage at an end, Dr. Harper began her new life in a new city, in a new job, as a newly single woman [1–3].

It was during this time of personal rupture that Dr. Harper began to truly see the connections between her own healing and that of her patients. In the ensuing years, as Dr. Harper learned to become an effective emergency physician, bringing insight and empathy to every patient encounter, she came to understand that each of us is broken; sometimes physically, oftentimes emotionally, and periodically psychically. This is the radical empathy that transforms good doctors into healers; the recognition that we are all wounded, all in need of mending.

Dr. Harper published her first book in July 2020 [1–3, 6]. "The Beauty in Breaking," arrived during a pandemic, during nationwide protests against police brutality, during a moment when the country was forced to confront long-ignored truths about racism and inequality. The timing was both fortuitous and terrible, a book about healing and brokenness released into a world coming apart at the seams.

"The Beauty in Breaking," is a New York Times bestseller in both hardcover and paperback editions [1, 4, 5]. "The Beauty in Breaking" is also a Los Angeles Times and Laura Bush Book Club pick, a Barnes & Noble Monthly Pick, a Book of the Month Club selection, and longlisted for the 2021 Andrew Carnegie Medals for Excellence in Nonfiction [4, 7]. These accolades speak to how Dr. Harper's story resonated with readers far beyond the medical community.

The book's critical reception has been remarkable [8]. The New York Times Book Review called it "Riveting, heartbreaking, sometimes difficult, always inspiring [3]." Ellen Pompeo described it as "An incredibly moving memoir about what it means to be a doctor [3]." Kerry Egan, author of "On Living," wrote: "'The Beauty in Breaking' takes us into the life in an emergency room—the drama, the adrenaline, the emotion—with such immediacy that I could not help but be completely enthralled by the individual stories of the patients that Michele Harper treats. But this powerful, poignant page-turner of a book also tells a much larger and universal story about how healing actually happens, not just for broken bodies but for broken hearts and souls [3]." This captures something essential about Dr. Harper's work; it is simultaneously a medical memoir, a personal narrative of survival, and a philosophical meditation on healing itself.

The book draws its title and central metaphor from the Japanese art of Kintsukuroi [1]. "In practicing the Japanese art of Kintsukuroi, one repairs broken pottery by filling in the cracks with gold, silver, or platinum. The choice to highlight the breaks with precious metals not only acknowledges them, but also pays tribute to the vessel that has been torn apart by the mutability of life. The previously broken object is considered more beautiful for its imperfections. In life, too, even greater brilliance can be found after mending," Dr. Harper writes [3]. This philosophy permeates every page of her memoir; the idea that our breaks, our traumas, our wounds can become sources of strength and beauty if we attend to them properly.

In this work, Dr. Harper weaves together patient stories with her own narrative of healing. Each chapter typically centers on a particular patient encounter that illuminates some aspect of brokenness and repair. She recalled in particular a woman covered with multiple stab wounds. Dr. Harper and her team stabilized her as she was bleeding, crying and in pain. "I wondered, What had brought her life to this point?" Dr. Harper asked. It turned out that an ex-partner had stabbed her. The medical intervention—stopping the bleeding, repairing tissue—is straightforward. But Dr. Harper asks deeper questions: What could I do as a physician and a human being to prevent this kind of violence from happening?

Another powerful story involves Dr. Harper's confrontation with systemic racism in real-time. Dr. Harper described an incident in which four police officers brought in a Black man and insisted he undergo an exam. They alleged he had swallowed a bag of drugs [2, 3]. While a nurse on the floor agreed with the officers and began to press for an exam, Dr. Harper began to ask the man questions. He firmly declined the exam, yet he appeared lucid, competent and sober as he denied the officers allegation.

What happened next demonstrates both Dr. Harper's courage and the complexity of practicing medicine while Black. A second-year resident training with her seemed to think she had more authority than Dr. Harper did. As Dr. Harper describes in her book, the resident threatened to report her for not going along with the police. Patients have rights, Dr. Harper explained. They have bodily autonomy. But he, unlike other people, didn't have rights in the moment before she intervened. Dr. Harper announced that she would not do the exam. And although her own resident questioned her decision, the hospitals ethics advisers backed Dr. Harpers decision.

When asked about this incident, Dr. Harper stated: "I know that she felt comfortable disregarding the rights of the patient and disregarding me. Why in her heart and mind did she do that? I don't know. Did the behavior exhibit flagrant unprofessionalism and quite frankly racism? Yes. Whether or not she understood that, whether or not she was consciously aware of her racism, I don't know." This is the exhausting reality for physicians of color; having to defend not just patients' rights but their own authority, their own expertise, their own humanity.

Dr. Harper is particularly attentive to how one of only about 2% of US physicians who are Black women navigates a system designed without her in mind [2]. Her advocacy for equity in medicine includes having served as chief medical advisor for Betr Remedies, a company dedicated to providing affordable medications to all [1]. Beyond direct patient care, Dr. Harper recognizes that healing requires addressing structural inequities, including medication access, which disproportionately affects vulnerable populations.

For her commitment to compassionate and equitable care in medicine, she was honored with the Gold Foundation National Humanism in Medicine Medal in 2022 [9]. This prestigious award recognizes physicians who exemplify the qualities of humanism in medicine: compassion, respect for human dignity, and dedication to the welfare of patients and society. The award underlines how Dr. Harper's benignant approach to medicine resonates with the profession's highest ideals.

Dr. Harper's ongoing work includes mentoring medical students and residents across the country and volunteering with STEM students from low-income communities [1]. She has also become a nationally recognized speaker whose work centers on individual healing and social justice [1, 10]. Dr. Harper has appeared nationwide, including at Yale University, the University of California San Diego, the University of Texas San Antonio, the Society of Academic Continuing Medical Education, and the American College of Surgeons, as well as Kaiser, Womanspace, T-Mobile, and Microsoft [1]. The breadth of these venues—from medical schools to corporations—demonstrates how her message transcends traditional medicine, speaking to anyone interested in healing, equity, and social justice.

Her media presence has been equally impressive. She has appeared as a commentator for MSNBC, NBC, ABC, and Cheddar networks, and on many popular podcasts [1]. As seen/heard on Fresh Air, The Daily Show with Trevor Noah, NBC Nightly News, MSNBC, Weekend Edition, and more [1, 11–14]. These appearances have brought her message to millions, using her platform to advocate for healthcare reform, racial justice, and provider wellness.

Dr. Harper's writing has also been featured in Zora and Elemental on Medium.com, and The Cut [1]. She is building a body of work beyond her memoir, continuing to explore themes of healing, identity, and justice through the written word. In 2023, Dr. Harper was awarded a MacDowell Fellowship in Literature [15]. During her time at MacDowell, she worked on her second book, a nonfiction memoir. MacDowell is one of the oldest and most prestigious artist residency programs in the United States, providing time and space for artists to work without distraction. That Dr. Harper was awarded this fellowship speaks to how seriously the literary world takes her work. Her second book is eagerly anticipated by readers who found healing and recognition in "The Beauty in Breaking."

Dr. Harper currently lives in the Washington, D.C. area, having returned to the city where she grew up [1]. She continues to practice medicine and is affiliated with Adventist HealthCare Fort Washington Medical Center and Fort Washington Medical Center in the Philadelphia area, maintaining her board certification in emergency medicine.

When asked by Annals of Emergency Medicine what she would like to tell an audience of emergency physicians, Dr. Harper responded: "This pandemic has been so painful; the loss of life, of income, the suffering. It has laid bare the failures of our system: there is no safety net. With record unemployment, so many people don't have insurance now. Health care providers hailed as heroes are being furloughed and fired, having their hours cut and their benefits cut. A demoralized work force is not going to be able to deliver the best care [2]."

But Dr. Harper doesn't stop at critique. "But this is an opportunity. If we could ignore these issues before, it is increasingly impossible to do so. We need to decide if we are going to go along with it or make change. This field isn't going to change itself. We need to decide how we want to practice medicine and take the steps to make it happen," she insists. This is Dr. Harper's approach in a nutshell; acknowledging pain and brokenness while insisting on the possibility of transformation [2].

Dr. Harper's impact on medicine extends beyond her clinical work or even her writing. She has helped shift the conversation about what it means to be a physician, a physician of color, and particularly a female physician. She has made visible the invisible; the microaggressions, the systemic racism, the emotional labor required to practice medicine while navigating discrimination. It is Dr. Harper's opinion and the American College of Emergency Physician's opinion that there is no role for bigotry in emergency medicine and in medicine period. Someone beholden to bigoted beliefs is not welcome in the field [1, 2].

This is the standard Dr. Harper holds herself and the profession to; a medicine that actively dismantles rather than perpetuates systems of oppression. "If that is the culture, then what is the nature of the care you expect to be given to patients? The culture needs to change," she said. This insistence on cultural transformation, on root-cause analysis rather than band-aid solutions, is what makes Dr. Harper's advocacy so powerful.

But perhaps her greatest contribution is showing us that our brokenness need not be hidden or denied but can become, through the right attention and care, a source of wisdom, empathy, and beauty. Like the pottery repaired with gold, we can be more beautiful for having been broken and mended. And in sharing that beauty with others—through patient care, through writing, through advocacy—we participate in the healing not just of individuals but of communities, systems, and perhaps even a nation.

References

1. Harper M. Michele Harper [Official website]. n.d. https://micheleharper.com/.
2. Kelly M. Annals Q & A with Dr. Michele Harper. Ann Emerg Med. 2020;76(5):A20–2. https://doi.org/10.1016/j.annemergmed.2020.10.001.
3. Harper M. The beauty in breaking. Riverhead Books; 2021. https://www.amazon.com/Beauty-Breaking-Memoir-Michele-Harper/dp/0525537392.
4. MacDowell. Michele Harper: Literature Fellow. 2023 https://www.macdowell.org/artists/michele-harper.
5. Penguin Random House. Michele Harper [Author page]. n.d. https://www.penguinrandomhouse.com/authors/2175605/michele-harper/.
6. Penguin Random House. The Beauty in Breaking by Michele Harper. 2020. https://www.penguinrandomhouse.com/books/580340/the-beauty-in-breaking-by-michele-harper/.
7. American Library Association. 2021 winners: Andrew Carnegie Medals for Excellence. Reference and User Services Association; 2021. https://www.ala.org/rusa/awards/carnegie-medals/2021-winners.
8. Kirkus Reviews. The Beauty in Breaking [Review]. 2020, March 29. https://www.kirkusreviews.com/book-reviews/michele-harper/the-beauty-in-breaking/.
9. Arnold P. Gold Foundation. Extraordinary GHHS leaders to be honored at the 2022 Gala. 2022. https://www.gold-foundation.org/newsroom/news/11-extraordinary-ghhs-leaders-to-be-honored-at-the-gold-gala/.
10. USC Health Sciences Campus. Michele Harper speaks to the Health Science Campus community. HSC News. 2022, November 14. https://hscnews.usc.edu/michele-harper-delivers-an-inspiring-lecture-to-the-health-sciences-campus-community.
11. Davies D. (Host). 'The Beauty in Breaking' chronicles chaos and healing in the emergency room [Audio podcast episode]. In Fresh Air. NPR. 2020, July 9. https://www.npr.org/2020/07/09/889407267/the-beauty-in-breaking-chronicles-chaos-and-healing-in-the-emergency-room.
12. Simon S. (Host). Dr. Michele Harper shares more than a decade of ER experience in new memoir [Audio podcast episode]. In Weekend Edition Saturday. NPR. 2020, July 4. https://www.npr.org/2020/07/04/887239274/dr-michele-harper-shares-more-than-a-decade-of-er-experience-in-new-memoir.
13. Ellison C. Watch: book club with Dr. Michele Harper. The Philadelphia Citizen. 2021, May 11. https://thephiladelphiacitizen.org/michele-harper-author-interview/.
14. Silverman E. (Host). Stories from the ER with Michele Harper, MD [Audio podcast episode]. In The Nocturnists. 2020. https://thenocturnists.org/podcast/micheleharper.
15. MacDowell. MacDowell awards spring-summer fellowships to 142 artists. 2023, February 17. https://www.macdowell.org/news/macdowell-awards-spring-summer-fellowships-to-142-artists.

Chapter 21
Danielle Ofri, MD, PhD

There is sacrifice in medicine—of time, of money, of comfort and sometimes of mental health. And we are humans at the end of the day, subject to the result of having made these valiant sacrifices, most of us in the early years of adulthood; hubris. We often enter medicine believing in our ability to battle disease and eradicate pathology, and very few things are as successful in disabusing this notion as caring for patients. We are reminded, time and time again, that often we are merely companions on a person's health journey, the route of which we may alter without ultimately changing the destination. Our patients humble us, with their non-classic presentations, their comorbidities, their fears, their internal and external struggles. These feelings of humility, some anxiety, mild to moderate terror, are felt while in training, but exacerbated by becoming an attending, when the proverbial buck stops with you. These emotions are dealt with by Dr. Danielle Ofri, from overcoming the mammoth that is medical school to approaching the colossus that is attendinghood. Her sketches demonstrate the chaos, grief, joy and pride of being inducted into the medical community, and then of being a minister of its teachings.

Dr. Danielle Ofri was born on August 22, 1965, in New York City [1, 2]. The city that never sleeps would become the backdrop for much of her medical career and the setting for many of the stories that would eventually comprise her literary work. Growing up in New York meant witnessing the extremes of urban life—wealth and poverty, health and sickness, community and isolation—all coexisting in the same dense geography.

She received an undergraduate degree in physiology from McGill University in Montreal in 1986 [2, 3]. From Montreal, she returned to her hometown for medical school, graduating from the New York University School of Medicine in 1993 with both an MD and a PhD in pharmacology [2, 4]. "When I started medical school, I had no idea that I would become a writer. I'd completed a PhD in the biochemistry of endorphin receptors, and planned to become a bench scientist with a once-a-week clinic to see patients," she would later reflect [5].

O. M. Cox, *The Pen, The Stethoscope, and The Scalpel*,
https://doi.org/10.1007/978-3-032-19406-0_21

But during residency, Dr. Ofri has said, something shifted; she fell in love with patient-care, and realized that she'd have to put bench research aside. This is a pivot many physician-scientists face; the pull between the laboratory and the bedside, between understanding disease in abstract molecular terms and treating actual suffering human beings. For Dr. Ofri, the choice was clear. The stories, the connections, and the humanity of medicine proved more compelling than the controlled environment of research.

She trained in internal medicine at Bellevue Hospital from 1993 to 1996 [2]. Bellevue, founded in 1736, is the oldest public hospital in the United States and one of the busiest urban hospitals in the country [1]. It is a place where the full spectrum of humanity passes through the emergency department doors. The poorest New Yorkers, the uninsured, the undocumented, those with nowhere else to go, Bellevue serves them all. It is also a teaching hospital, training generations of physicians in the realities of urban medicine. Training at Bellevue is not for the faint of heart. The patient population is complex; multiple comorbidities, language barriers, social determinants of health that complicate every treatment plan. The volume is relentless. The resources, while substantial, are stretched thin. Yet for those who train there, Bellevue becomes more than a hospital; it becomes a crucible where doctors are forged through fire.

After completing residency, Dr. Ofri took some time to travel [3]. She spent 18 months on the road, working occasional medical temp-jobs to earn money, and then exploring Latin America for as long as her money would last. This period of wandering, of stepping away from the intensity of residency, proved crucial. It was during these travels, during this first true break from medicine, that she started writing down the stories of her medical training at Bellevue Hospital. At the time, she had no intentions about a book, or publishing.

But those stories, once captured on paper, demanded to be shared. These essays were published in literary journals and eventually formed the basis of her first book, "Singular Intimacies: Becoming a Doctor at Bellevue," originally published in 2003 [1, 6]. The book traces her experiences in medical school and residency at an inner-city hospital, and it resonated deeply with both medical and general audiences. The New England Journal of Medicine's Robert S. Schwartz observed: "Ofri is a gifted writer. Her vignettes ring with truth, and for any physician or patient who knows the dramas of a big-city hospital they will evoke tears, laughter, and memories [1]." This is high praise from one of medicine's most prestigious journals; recognition that Dr. Ofri had found a way to capture the essence of medical training in prose that was both literary and authentic. An essay from the book, "Merced," was chosen by Stephen Jay Gould for Best American Essays 2002, and was awarded the Editor's Prize for Nonfiction by The Missouri Review [3, 7].

"Singular Intimacies" is so compelling in part because of its setting; Bellevue itself is a character in these stories, with its long history, its institutional memory, its role as safety net for the city [1, 6]. A large part of the book's success, though, is due to Dr. Ofri's stark honesty about the uncertainty, fear, and doubt that accompany medical training. She writes about struggling to arrange heart surgery for a veteran plagued with drug-addiction, dealing with the suicide of a demanding hospital supervisor, hearing a French woman's dying request to have her body flown back to Paris [1, 6].

These are not triumphant tales of medical heroism. They are stories of human connection in the face of suffering, of small victories and devastating losses, of learning to be a doctor by being present with patients in their most vulnerable moments. "Ofri relates each transforming experience in prose so powerful in its lucidity and quest for truth that it arouses both tears and wonder," Booklist critic Donna Seaman wrote [3].

Her second book, "Incidental Findings: Lessons from my Patients in the Art of Medicine," was published in 2005 [1, 8]. This collection explores the subject of teaching medicine to the next generation of physicians, as well as Dr. Ofri's experiences as a "locum tenens" physician in small town America. The book also includes something unexpected; Dr. Ofri writing about her own experience being a patient. Her essay "Living Will," was selected by Susan Orlean for Best American Essays 2005 [1, 7]. The essay "Common Ground," was selected by Oliver Sacks for Best American Science Writing 2003 and granted an honorable mention by Anne Fadiman in Best American Essays 2004 [1, 3, 7].

In 2010, she released "Medicine in Translation: Journeys with My Patients," her third book [1, 5]. It discusses immigration and health care; two topics that dominated public discourse in 2010 and remain urgent today. Dr. Ofri explores the cultural challenges in medicine, and chronicles the experiences of immigrants and Americans in the U.S. health care system. At Bellevue, where the patient population reflects New York City's incredible diversity, language barriers and cultural differences are not occasional complications but daily realities. Dr. Ofri writes about navigating these challenges, and about the ways translation—both linguistic and cultural—shapes medical care.

Her fourth book, "What Doctors Feel: How Emotions Affect the Practice of Medicine," was published in 2013 [1, 9]. This book examines the emotional side of medicine that impacts patient care. "Fear is a primal emotion in medicine. Every doctor can tell you of times when she or he was terrified; most can list more episodes than you might wish to hear," Dr. Ofri writes. "It may be sublimated at times, it may wax and wane, but the fear of harming your patients never departs; it is inextricably linked to the practice of medicine [9]."

This acknowledgment of fear, of the emotional weight physicians carry, was radical when the book was published and remains as poignant today. Medical culture traditionally demands stoicism, demands that doctors suppress their emotions in service of clinical objectivity. But Dr. Ofri argues convincingly that emotions are not impediments to good medicine, they are integral to it. "Empathy, the ability to identify with someone else's suffering, is certainly a prerequisite for a genuine apology," she writes [9].

Dr. Ofri's fifth book, "What Patients Say, What Doctors Hear," was published in 2017 [1, 10]. It explores the doctor-patient conversation as the most powerful tool in medicine. Though the gulf between what patients say and what doctors hear is often wide, Dr. Ofri proves that it doesn't have to be. Through powerfully resonant human stories, she explores the high-stakes world of doctor-patient communication that we all must navigate. Reporting on the latest research studies and interviewing scholars, doctors, and patients, she reveals how better communication can lead to better health for all of us. The book has been translated into multiple languages—Japanese, Chinese, and Italian—with a Spanish edition published subsequently. This international reach demonstrates how the challenges of doctor-patient communication transcend cultural boundaries.

Her sixth and most recent book, "When We Do Harm: A Doctor Confronts Medical Error," was published in 2020 [1, 11]. This book places the issues of medical error and patient safety front and center in our national healthcare conversation. Medical mistakes are more pervasive than we think, Dr. Ofri describes. Patients enter the medical system with faith that they will receive the best care possible, so when things go wrong, it becomes a profound and painful breach.

The book's timing was significant; published at the beginning of the COVID-19 pandemic, it was a time when the healthcare system was pushed to its limits and medical errors became more likely due to overwhelmed staff, shortages of equipment, and rapidly evolving treatment protocols. "What makes this book special is Ofri's perceptive and compassionate nature; she sees her own patients as real people and is candid with readers about her concerns and vulnerabilities…Thorough analysis of a challenging problem executed with a personal touch that makes it highly readable," according to Kirkus Reviews in a starred review [12]. "An essential read for anyone involved or interested in the care of patients," noted Booklist [1].

Beyond her books, Dr. Ofri has maintained a prolific presence in medical and mainstream media. She writes regularly for The New York Times health section about medicine and the doctor-patient connection. Her writing also appears in The New Yorker, The Atlantic, The Lancet, The New England Journal of Medicine, the Los Angeles Times, the Washington Post, Slate Magazine, CNN, and on National Public Radio [1, 2].

In 2000, Dr. Ofri co-founded the Bellevue Literary Review, the first literary magazine to arise from a hospital setting [13]. She remains Editor-in-Chief of this now-independent nonprofit literary arts organization [1, 2, 13]. The Bellevue Literary Review publishes works of fiction, nonfiction, and poetry "that touch upon relationships to the human body, illness, health and healing." It is now considered the preeminent journal in its field and received a prestigious Whiting Award [14]. The journal has published work by established authors and emerging voices, contributing to the field of medical humanities and expanding our understanding of how literature can illuminate medical experience.

Dr. Ofri returned to Bellevue Hospital as an attending physician in 1998, where she continues to teach and practice medicine as a primary care internist [1, 2]. She is also a clinical professor of medicine at New York University School of Medicine [2]. For over two decades, she has maintained this triple practice—clinician, teacher, and writer—each role informing and enriching the others.

Her recognition by the medical community has been extensive. She is a Fellow of the American College of Physicians and has been elevated to "Master" status, an honor reserved for physicians who have made outstanding contributions to internal medicine [1]. She received the McGovern Award from the American Medical

Writers Association for "preeminent contributions to medical communication [1]." She has also received an honorary doctorate of humane letters from Curry College in Boston [1].

Most recently, her accolades have multiplied; the 2023 Guggenheim Fellowship from the John Simon Guggenheim Memorial Foundation [4, 15], the 2023 Nicholas E. Davies Memorial Scholar Award for Scholarly Activities in the Humanities and History of Medicine from the American College of Physicians [16], the 2022 National Humanism in Medicine Medal from the Gold Foundation [17], and the 2020 Global Listening Legend Award [1]. The Arnold P. Gold Foundation recognized Dr. Ofri as "one of the foremost voices in the medical world today, speaking passionately about the doctor-patient relationship and sustaining humanity in healthcare [17]." Dr. Ofri has also given TED talks on "Deconstructing Perfection" and "Fear: A Necessary Emotion," and has performed stories for The Moth. She is featured in the documentaries Why Doctors Write and White Coat Rebels [18]. These honors recognize not just her writing but her advocacy for humanistic medicine, for listening to patients, for bringing empathy back to the center of medical practice.

Dr. Ofri lives in New York City with her three children and studies cello [1]. In lieu of going to the gym, she spends most evenings wrestling with the Bach cello suites, routinely bested by a guy who's been dead for 270 years, as she wryly notes [19]. She strives for a serene, uncluttered life of Zen, but has teenagers instead.

Dr. Ofri reminds us that it remains possible to maintain that connection even in the busiest, most resource-constrained settings. She did it at Bellevue, caring for the poorest and most marginalized New Yorkers. She continues to do it, seeing patients while also teaching, writing, editing, speaking, and raising three children. If she can preserve the humanity of medicine while juggling all these demands, perhaps there's hope for all of us. Her work also reminds us that telling our stories matters. The stories of our training, our patients, our mistakes, our triumphs. These stories teach us, console us, and connect us to one another.

References

1. Ofri D. Danielle Ofri [Official website]. n.d. https://danielleofri.com/.
2. NYU Grossman School of Medicine. Danielle Ofri, MD, PhD. n.d. https://med.nyu.edu/faculty/danielle-ofri.
3. Encyclopedia.com. Ofri, Danielle. n.d. https://www.encyclopedia.com/arts/educational-magazines/ofri-danielle.
4. Doximity. Dr. Danielle Ofri, MD—New York, NY | Internal Medicine. n.d. https://www.doximity.com/pub/danielle-ofri-md.
5. Ofri D. Medicine in translation: journeys with my patients. Boston: Beacon Press; 2010.
6. Ofri D. Singular intimacies: becoming a doctor at Bellevue. Boston: Beacon Press; 2003.
7. Ofri D. Danielle Ofri M.D., Ph.D. Psychology Today. n.d. https://www.psychologytoday.com/us/contributors/danielle-ofri-md-phd.
8. Ofri D. Incidental findings: lessons from my patients in the art of medicine. Boston: Beacon Press; 2005.

9. Ofri D. What doctors feel: how emotions affect the practice of medicine. Boston: Beacon Press; 2013.
10. Ofri D. What patients say, what doctors hear. Boston: Beacon Press; 2017.
11. Ofri D. When we do harm: a doctor confronts medical error. Boston: Beacon Press; 2020.
12. Kirkus Reviews. When we do harm [Book review]. 2020, January 15. https://www.kirkusreviews.com/book-reviews/danielle-ofri-3/when-we-do-harm/.
13. Bellevue Literary Review. Home. n.d. https://blreview.org.
14. Whiting Foundation. Bellevue literary review. n.d. https://www.whiting.org/content/bellevue-literary-review.
15. NYU News. Five NYU faculty awarded 2023 Guggenheim Fellowships. 2023, April. https://www.nyu.edu/about/news-publications/news/2023/april/five-nyu-faculty-awarded-2023-guggenheim-fellowships.html.
16. American College of Physicians. ACP announces 2022–23 recipients of Masterships and National Awards. 2023. https://www.acponline.org/about-acp/awards-masterships-and-competitions/acp-announces-2022-23-recipients-of-masterships-and-national-awards.
17. Arnold P. Gold Foundation. Gold Foundation to honor four inspiring leaders with 2022 National Humanism in Medicine Medals. 2022. https://www.gold-foundation.org/newsroom/news/gold-foundation-to-honor-four-inspiring-leaders-with-2022-national-humanism-in-medicine-medals/.
18. Ofri D. NPR [Tag archive]. Danielle Ofri. n.d. https://danielleofri.com/tag/npr/.
19. American Medical Women's Association. Meet the author: Dr. Danielle Ofri speaks on her new book, When we do harm. 2020, April 22. https://amwa-doc.org/news/meet-the-author-dr-danielle-ofri-speaks-on-her-new-book-when-we-do-harm/.

Chapter 22
Julie Holland, MD

In psychiatry, we learn to understand criteria for diagnoses through the use of the DSM (Diagnostic and Statistical Manual of Mental Disorders), a pocket copy of which we were provided at the start of our clinical year rotations. Much of appreciating the various ways a mind may be injured, involves recognizing its normal patterns of function. Physiology and then pathology, as with all parts of medicine. Yet, unlike the Renal or Endocrine systems, the testing for pathology, within psychiatry, occurs over hours, and not minutes; face-to-face and not via a lab close to the patient's home. And while criteria are universally accepted for categorizing kidney failure or hyperthyroidism, the guidelines within psychiatry do not, almost necessarily, apply to every patient. The variety in human behavior, it turns out, is too vast to fit into one book, even one with over a thousand pages, such as the DSM-5-TR. In Dr. Julie Holland's work, we are given the opportunity to explore this variety, while simultaneously reflecting on our role as arbiters of mental health. Whether we *should* take on this mantle, what responsibility this entails and how we might optimize the interactions that characterize this role.

Dr. Julie Holland was born on December 13, 1965, in New York City, though she would spend her formative years in Framingham, Massachusetts, a suburb of Boston [1, 2]. From an early age, Dr. Holland demonstrated an intellectual curiosity that would eventually draw her toward the intersection of brain science and human behavior. When she arrived at the University of Pennsylvania for her undergraduate education, she found a program perfectly suited to her emerging interests: the Biological Basis of Behavior, an interdisciplinary major combining the study of psychology and neural sciences [1, 2]. Within this program, Holland developed a particular concentration in psychopharmacology, a focus that would define her career and establish her as one of the most prominent voices in American psychiatry.

It was during her college years that Dr. Holland first demonstrated the intellectual audacity that would become her hallmark. She authored an extensive research paper on MDMA, the compound commonly known as Ecstasy, at a time when the

O. M. Cox, *The Pen, The Stethoscope, and The Scalpel*,
https://doi.org/10.1007/978-3-032-19406-0_22

substance was transitioning from therapeutic tool to criminalized street drug [1, 2]. This undergraduate work would prove remarkably prescient; it became the foundation for her 2001 book, "Ecstasy: The Complete Guide: A Comprehensive Look at the Risks and Benefits of MDMA," a scholarly work that examined the substance with scientific rigor rather than moral panic [1, 3]. In an era dominated by Just Say No rhetoric, Dr. Holland was already asking more nuanced questions about consciousness, medicine, and the arbitrary lines society draws between legitimate treatment and forbidden experience.

After completing her undergraduate degree, Dr. Holland pursued her medical education at Temple University School of Medicine, receiving her MD in 1992 [1]. Her residency at Mount Sinai Hospital in New York would prove transformative. There, she served as Chief Resident of the Schizophrenia Research Ward, a position that placed her at the frontier of psychiatric treatment for one of the most severe and misunderstood mental illnesses [1]. As principal investigator in a research study examining a new medication for schizophrenia, Dr. Holland distinguished herself among her peers, earning the National Institute of Mental Health Outstanding Resident Award in 1994 [1]. This recognition marked her as a physician of exceptional promise, one whose talents extended beyond clinical care into the realm of research and innovation.

But it was her next position that would define Dr. Holland's public identity and provide the raw material for her most celebrated work. In 1996, she accepted a position as an attending psychiatrist in the Comprehensive Psychiatric Emergency Program at Bellevue Hospital in New York City. Specifically, the weekend night shift [1, 4]. She would hold this position for 9 years, until 2005, spending her Saturday and Sunday nights as the physician in charge of admissions to one of America's most storied psychiatric emergency rooms.

To understand the significance of this position, one must understand Bellevue itself. Established in 1736, Bellevue Hospital is the oldest public hospital in the United States; a six-bed infirmary that opened on the second floor of the New York City Almshouse just 4 years after George Washington's birth and 40 years before the Declaration of Independence [5, 6]. Over nearly three centuries, Bellevue has served as an incubator for major innovations in public health, medical science, and medical education. It established America's first maternity ward, nursing school, on-site medical college, emergency service, psychiatric ward, ambulance corps, and pathology department. The hospital has confronted every major epidemic in American history: cholera in 1832, typhus in 1847, tuberculosis throughout the nineteenth century, AIDS in the 1980s, and the Ebola scare of 2014 [5, 6].

Yet for all its medical achievements, Bellevue became infamous in the public consciousness for its psychiatric wing. The hospital's name became a byword for insanity itself, a cultural shorthand for mental illness so entrenched that generations of New York parents threatened misbehaving children with being sent there. This reputation crystallized in 1887 when the pioneering journalist Nellie Bly feigned mental illness to gain admission to Bellevue, subsequently documenting the barbaric conditions she witnessed at the Blackwell's Island asylum where patients were transferred. Her exposé, *Ten Days in a Madhouse*, became a bestseller and forever linked Bellevue to the treatment—and mistreatment—of the mentally ill in the American imagination [7].

This was the institution where Dr. Julie Holland chose to spend her weekends for nearly a decade. As she would later write, Bellevue's psychiatric emergency room was a place where she encountered the spectrum of human mental distress: the psychotic, the suicidal, the violent, the confused, the addicted, the homeless, and the desperate [4]. Prisoners in chains arrived alongside battered women. The delusional shared space with those feigning symptoms to secure a warm bed and a hot meal. Serial killers passed through the same doors as subway conductors traumatized by witnessing passengers pushed onto tracks. In this den of human suffering and resilience, Dr. Holland developed her understanding of mental illness, and of herself as a healer [1].

The memoir that emerged from this experience, "Weekends at Bellevue: Nine Years on the Night Shift at the Psych ER," published in 2009, became a nationally bestselling book that introduced Dr. Holland to a broader audience [1, 8, 9]. Critics praised it as a work that combined the page-turning immediacy of a television medical drama with a fascinating glimpse into the inner lives of physicians who struggle to maintain perspective in a world where sanity is in the eye of the beholder. Andrew Weil, the renowned integrative medicine physician, called it "an extraordinary insider's look at the typical days and nights of that most extraordinary place, written with a rare combination of toughness, tenderness, and outrageous humor [8]." The neurosurgeon Katrina Firlik, author of "Another Day in the Frontal Lobe," described it as "a gem of a memoir" that "leaves deep tracks in even the healthiest of minds [8]."

What characterized Dr. Holland's memoir amongst other medical narratives at the time, was her unadorned honesty about her own evolution as a physician. She documented her transformation from a 30-year-old with a "macho swagger" and a tough-girl attitude to what she described as a "working mother of two with a heart of mush [8]." She acknowledged the defensive cynicism that helped her cope with daily exposure to human tragedy, and she chronicled the moments that cracked that defense, including her first patient suicide, which taught her that her obligation as a psychiatrist extended beyond alleviating the patient's pain to preventing the grief of those who would be left behind. As she wrote, "Doctors are supposed to alleviate pain. Psychiatrists are meant not only to soothe the despair and hopelessness that a depressed person experiences, but also, I have come to realize, to prevent the pain of the ones who would be left behind [8]."

The success of "Weekends at Bellevue" established Dr. Holland as a public intellectual, a physician whose voice extended beyond the clinical setting into the broader cultural conversation about mental health [1, 8, 10]. This platform enabled her to pursue her longstanding interest in substances that existed in a gray zone between medicine and criminality. In 2010, she edited and published "The Pot Book: A Complete Guide to Cannabis," a comprehensive edited volume that explored the role of cannabis in medicine, politics, history, and society [11]. As with her earlier book on MDMA, "The Pot Book," was structured as a nonprofit project, with proceeds funding therapeutic research rather than enriching the author [1, 2]. Dr. Holland assembled contributions from leading experts including Lester

Grinspoon, Rick Doblin, and Michael Pollan, creating a resource that examined marijuana with the scientific seriousness it had long been denied by both drug warriors and counterculture advocates [11].

Throughout this period, Dr. Holland maintained her visibility as a media commentator on issues related to mental illness and drug use. She appeared on The Today Show more than 25 times and became a regular presence on CNN, most notably in Dr. Sanjay Gupta's documentary series *Weed* [2]. She was quoted as an expert in Time, Harper's, Slate, the Los Angeles Times, and The Wall Street Journal [1, 12]. This media presence reflected both her expertise and her gift for communicating complex scientific and medical information to general audiences, a talent that would prove central to her most commercially successful work.

That work arrived in 2015 with "Moody Bitches: The Truth About the Drugs You're Taking, the Sleep You're Missing, the Sex You're Not Having, and What's Really Making You Crazy [13, 14]." The provocatively titled book became a New York Times bestseller and was subsequently translated into 11 languages, introducing Dr. Holland's ideas to readers around the world [1, 13, 14]. In it, she offered a feminist critique of the psychiatric establishment's treatment of women, arguing that the natural moodiness and emotional sensitivity that characterize female psychology had been pathologized and medicated rather than understood and honored [13, 14].

Dr. Holland's central argument was both scientifically grounded and culturally provocative. She noted that at least one in four women in America now takes a psychiatric medication, compared with one in seven men. Rather than accepting this disparity as evidence that women are inherently more mentally ill than men, Dr. Holland proposed an alternative interpretation: women's emotions were being medicated away because they made others uncomfortable. "We are not men," she wrote. "We are women. We feel more deeply, express our emotions more frequently, and get moody monthly. It's normal. It's nature's way. And we don't necessarily have to medicate away the essence of who we are to make others more comfortable [13, 14]."

The book arrived at a cultural moment primed for its message. In February 2015, Dr. Holland published an op-ed in The New York Times titled "Medicating Women's Feeling," that distilled her argument to its essence [15]. "Women's emotionality is a sign of health, not disease; it is a source of power," she wrote. "But we are under constant pressure to restrain our emotional lives. We have been taught to apologize for our tears, to suppress our anger and to fear being called hysterical. The pharmaceutical industry plays on that fear, targeting women in a barrage of advertising on daytime talk shows and in magazines [15]." The piece sparked widespread discussion and debate, bringing academic feminist critiques of psychiatry into mainstream conversation.

"Moody Bitches," offered practical guidance alongside its cultural critique [13, 14]. Dr. Holland provided detailed information about psychiatric medications and their effects on women's bodies, discussed the connection between food and mood, and offered advice on sleep, exercise, and sexual health. She explored natural therapies and lifestyle modifications that could address many of the symptoms for which women were being prescribed powerful psychotropic drugs. Reviewers compared the book to "Our Bodies, Ourselves," the landmark 1970 feminist health guide, suggesting that Dr. Holland had created a similarly transformative resource for a new generation. Douglas Rushkoff, author of "Present Shock," called it "the most important book on being a woman since 'Our Bodies, Our Selves' [13, 14]."

The book's impact extended beyond individual readers to influence broader conversations about women's mental health care. Dr. Holland challenged the pharmaceutical industry's targeting of women through advertising campaigns that presented normal emotional experiences as pathologies requiring medication. She postulated that women's higher rates of prescription psychiatric medications reflected a cultural discomfort with female emotion and a medical establishment too quick to reach for the prescription pad. Her critique resonated particularly strongly with women who had felt pathologized by medical professionals for expressing emotions that struck them as entirely appropriate responses to their circumstances.

While building her public platform, Dr. Holland continued her work at the frontier of psychedelic research. She became a medical advisor to MAPS, the Multidisciplinary Association for Psychedelic Studies, serving as medical monitor for several clinical studies examining the efficacy of MDMA-assisted psychotherapy in the treatment of post-traumatic stress disorder [1, 2]. This work placed her at the center of what many observers consider a renaissance in psychiatric treatment; the return of psychedelic substances to legitimate medical research after decades of prohibition and stigma.

The clinical trials Dr. Holland helped oversee produced remarkable results. In studies involving military veterans, firefighters, and police officers—populations with high rates of treatment-resistant PTSD—MDMA-assisted psychotherapy showed significant efficacy [1, 2]. The research suggested that carefully administered psychedelic experiences, conducted in therapeutic settings with trained facilitators, could help patients process trauma that had proven impervious to conventional treatments [16]. Holland's involvement lent medical credibility to work that had previously been dismissed as countercultural fantasy, helping to shift the conversation around psychedelics from prohibition to potential.

This research informed Dr. Holland's most recent book, "Good Chemistry: The Science of Connection, from Soul to Psychedelics," published in June 2020 [17, 18]. The book arrived at a moment of unprecedented social isolation; the COVID-19 pandemic had forced millions into quarantine, making questions of human connection urgently relevant. Dr. Holland argued that Americans were suffering from an epidemic of disconnection that antidepressants and social media could not fix. This state of isolation, she wrote, puts us in "fight or flight mode," disrupting sleep, metabolism, and libido while fostering paranoia toward others [17, 18].

The timing of the book's publication proved both fortuitous; as the pandemic forced people into physical isolation, Dr. Holland's arguments about the essential nature of human connection gained new urgency [19]. She drew on research showing that social isolation carries health risks comparable to smoking 15 cigarettes daily, that the opioid epidemic itself could be understood partly as a symptom of disconnection, and that the digital connections offered by social media often exacerbate rather than alleviate loneliness [20–22]. Against this backdrop of isolation, she offered psychedelic medicines as one potential pathway back to connection; not as a cure-all, but as tools that, when used appropriately, could help catalyze the neurochemical and psychological changes necessary for genuine bonding.

"Good Chemistry" explores the neuroscience of connection, focusing particularly on oxytocin, the hormone and neurotransmitter that enables humans to trust and bond [17, 18]. Dr. Holland examined various pathways to accessing what she called "feel-good chemistry": conscious breathing, sex, meditation, group activities, and psychedelic medicines. She conveyed what Kirkus Reviews described as "great excitement and marvelous anecdotes about the prospects of the psychedelic pharmacopeia," while grounding her enthusiasm in scientific research and clinical experience [17, 18].

Elizabeth Lesser, cofounder of the Omega Institute and bestselling author, praised Dr. Holland for combining "science with soul and cutting-edge research with compelling stories of lives changed and psyches mended, in a book that is helpful, moving, and highly relevant to our disconnected and anxious times [17, 18]." Gabor Maté, the renowned trauma expert, called the book "reader-friendly" in the truest sense, noting that "it befriends us, the readers. It speaks to us plainly and gently, keeps us company, and offers practical antidotes to the estrangement from ourselves and others so endemic in modern society [17, 18]."

Today, Dr. Julie Holland maintains a private psychiatric practice in midtown Manhattan, where she continues to see patients and prescribe medications when appropriate while also exploring alternatives to pharmaceutical intervention [1]. She remains active as a medical advisor to MAPS and other organizations working to bring psychedelic-assisted therapy into mainstream medicine [2]. She has worked for decades on drug policy reform based on harm reduction principles, advocating for an approach that prioritizes public health over criminalization. Her work as a forensic consultant on drug-related cases brings her expertise into legal settings, where she provides testimony on matters involving PCP, MDMA, and other substances [1]. This work reflects her status as one of America's foremost experts on street drugs and intoxication states; knowledge earned through her years in Bellevue's psychiatric emergency room and her ongoing research into the effects of various substances on human consciousness and behavior.

The DSM provides us with categories and criteria, but as Dr. Holland's words reminds us, the human beings we treat will always exceed those categories. Our task as physicians is not merely to classify and medicate but to witness, to understand, and ultimately to help our patients find their way back to connection; with themselves, with others, and with the splendor and wonderment that exists everywhere we choose to see it. In the tradition of physician-writers who use the pen to extend their healing influence beyond the clinic, Dr. Julie Holland has written herself into the history of American medicine and literature alike.

References

1. Holland J. Julie Holland, M.D. [Official website]. n.d. https://drholland.com/.
2. MAPS Public Benefit Corporation. Julie Holland, M.D. [Staff profile]. n.d. https://mapspublicbenefit.com/staff/julie-holland-m-d/.
3. Holland J, editor. Ecstasy: the complete guide: a comprehensive look at the risks and benefits of MDMA. Park Street Press; 2001. https://www.simonandschuster.com/books/Ecstasy-The-Complete-Guide/Julie-Holland/9780892818570.
4. Psychotherapy.net. Weekends at Bellevue excerpt. n.d. https://www.psychotherapy.net/article/weekends-at-bellevue.
5. NYC Health + Hospitals. Bellevue history. n.d. https://www.nychealthandhospitals.org/bellevue/history/.
6. Fiani B, Covarrubias C, Jarrah R, Kondilis A, Doan TM. Bellevue Hospital, the oldest public health center in The United States of America. World Neurosurg. 2022;167:57–61. https://doi.org/10.1016/j.wneu.2022.08.088.
7. Bly N. Ten days in a mad-house. CreateSpace; 2011. https://www.amazon.com/Ten-Days-Mad-House-Nellie-Bly/dp/146369539X.
8. Holland J. Weekends at Bellevue. Bantam; 2009. https://www.amazon.com/Weekends-Bellevue-Years-Night-Shift/dp/0553386522.
9. Holland J. Weekends at Bellevue: nine years on the night shift at the psych ER. Bantam Books; 2009. https://www.penguinrandomhouse.com/books/81793/weekends-at-bellevue-by-julie-holland/9780553386523/.
10. Kirkus Reviews. Weekends at Bellevue [Book review]. 2009, July 15. https://www.kirkusreviews.com/book-reviews/julie-holland/weekends-at-bellevue/.
11. Holland J, editor. The pot book: a complete guide to cannabis. Park Street Press; 2010. https://www.simonandschuster.com/books/The-Pot-Book/Julie-Holland/9781594773686.
12. Amazon. Julie Holland M.D.: books, biography, latest update. n.d. https://www.amazon.com/stores/author/B002G5S71Q.
13. Holland J. Moody bitches: the truth about the drugs you're taking, the sleep you're missing, the sex you're not having, and what's really making you crazy. Penguin Books; 2015. https://www.amazon.com/Moody-Bitches-Taking-Missing-Having/dp/0143107909.
14. Holland J. Moody bitches: the truth about the drugs you're taking, the sleep you're missing, the sex you're not having, and what's really making you crazy. Penguin Press; 2015. https://www.penguinrandomhouse.com/books/314941/moody-bitches-by-julie-holland-md/.
15. Holland J. Medicating women's feelings [Op-ed]. The New York Times. 2015, February 28. https://www.nytimes.com/2015/03/01/opinion/sunday/medicating-womens-feelings.html.
16. Mithoefer MC, Mithoefer AT, Feduccia AA, Jerome L, Wagner M, Wymer J, Holland J, Hamilton S, Yazar-Klosinski B, Emerson A, Doblin R. 3,4-methylenedioxymethamphetamine (MDMA)-assisted psychotherapy for post-traumatic stress disorder in military veterans, firefighters, and police officers: a randomised, double-blind, dose-response, phase 2 clinical trial. Lancet Psychiatry. 2018;5(6):486–97. https://doi.org/10.1016/S2215-0366(18)30135-4.
17. Holland J. Good chemistry: the science of connection, from soul to psychedelics. HarperWave. 2020. https://www.harperwave.com/book/9780062862884/Good-Chemistry-Julie-Holland/.
18. Holland J. Good chemistry: the science of connection, from soul to psychedelics. HarperWave. 2020. https://www.amazon.com/Good-Chemistry-Science-Connection-Psychedelics/dp/006286288X.
19. Matos M, McEwan K, Kanovský M, Halamová J, Steindl SR, Ferreira N, Linharelhos M, Rijo D, Asano K, Vilas SP, Márquez MG, Gregório S, Brito-Pons G, Lucena-Santos P, Oliveira MDS, Souza EL, Llobenes L, Gumiy N, Costa MI, Habib N, Gilbert P. The role of social connection on the experience of COVID-19 related post-traumatic growth and stress. PLoS One. 2021;16(12):e0261384. https://doi.org/10.1371/journal.pone.0261384.

20. Holt-Lunstad J, Smith TB, Layton JB. Social relationships and mortality risk: a meta-analytic review. PLoS Med. 2010;7(7):e1000316. https://doi.org/10.1371/journal.pmed.1000316.
21. Christie NC. The role of social isolation in opioid addiction. Soc Cogn Affect Neurosci. 2021;16(7):645–56. https://doi.org/10.1093/scan/nsab029.
22. Koh GK, Ow Yong JQY, Lee ARYB, Ong BSY, Yau CE, Ho CSH, Goh YS. Social media use and its impact on adults' mental health and well-being: a scoping review. Worldviews Evid-Based Nurs. 2024;21(4):345–94. https://doi.org/10.1111/wvn.12727.

Chapter 23
Esther Sternberg, MD

I recall being advised to ask about Wellness Initiatives during my residency interviews, and then considering that Wellness, as a concept, held such a broad definition that initiatives to promote it varied from the inclusion of windows in workrooms to sugary treat deliveries. The only consensus seemed to be that there was a tangible gain and loss in productivity depending on how trainees felt. Wellness appeared to be the intersection of protected mental health and nurtured physical body; it was tied to individual sense of self, personal ranks of priority, and how best both are cultivated. It was impossible to develop a One Size Fits All model for successfully achieving wellness in residency classes that sometimes numbered above 100, but it was important to understand that maintaining wellness was key to preserving the health of each new class of physicians. Understanding how our environments, physical and social, can improve or stagnate physician clinical and scholastic growth was at the root of these discussions on wellness. Dr. Esther Sternberg understood the critical role of the environment on the body and has used her career to spearhead systemic change in how we approach wellness. Not simply as a checklist of items to offer trainees, or patients, but as intrinsic to the foundation of good health.

Dr. Esther Sternberg was born in 1951 in Montreal, Canada, into a family where science and medicine were not abstractions but daily realities [1, 2]. Her father, Dr. Joseph Sternberg, was a physician-scientist and a pioneer in the fields of radiation biology and nuclear medicine. Her aunt was a professor of physiology at McGill University. Surrounded by scientists and physicians from her earliest memories, Esther took for granted the lifestyle of the physician-researcher-scientist, though she did not initially imagine herself following the same path. As a teenager, she was interested in many aspects of biology; she recalls reading a three-volume book on worms in junior high, nurturing interests in paleontology, dinosaurs, and archeology. The idea of becoming a doctor did not seem inevitable [2].

It was her high school guidance counselor who first suggested she apply to McGill University's seven-year medical program, which accepted students directly from high school for an accelerated undergraduate and medical education. Initially

O. M. Cox, *The Pen, The Stethoscope, and The Scalpel*,
https://doi.org/10.1007/978-3-032-19406-0_23

reluctant, Sternberg was eventually persuaded to apply [2]. When she imagined herself graduating from medical school, she later admitted, she visualized herself transforming into Dr. Kildare, the handsome, heroic physician from the eponymous NBC medical drama airing at the time [1]. She did not have a female physician role model, and without realizing it, her mental image of a doctor remained distinctly male. It was a subtle but telling indication of the world she was about to enter, and the challenges she would face in carving her own identity within it.

Dr. Sternberg received her Bachelor of Science degree with Great Distinction from McGill University in 1972, and, her medical degree from McGill's Faculty of Medicine in 1974 [3, 4]. She completed her residency in internal medicine and her fellowship in rheumatology at McGill, developing an expertise in autoimmune diseases that would become foundational to her later research [3, 4]. After her training, she was appointed as an associate of the prestigious Howard Hughes Medical Institute and an instructor in medicine at Washington University and Barnes Hospital in St. Louis [2]. There, she entered general practice, and from 1984 to 1986 served as an attending physician at Barnes Hospital. Her patient interactions were described as rewarding and would serve as the pathway toward her research endeavors [2].

In 1986, Dr. Sternberg joined the National Institutes of Health, where she would spend the next 26 years as a senior scientist and section chief [2]. At the National Institute of Mental Health, she served as Chief of the Section on Neuroendocrine Immunology and Behavior, Director of the Integrative Neural Immune Program, and Co-Chair of the NIH Intramural Program on Research on Women's Health. Her research focused on the interactions between the central nervous system and the immune system, a field that, when she entered it, was still in its infancy and regarded with skepticism by many in mainstream medicine [2].

The prevailing view in the scientific community at the time held that the immune system was autonomous, a self-contained defense mechanism operating independently of the brain and its emotional processing. This separation had deep roots in the history of Western medicine, which had long divided the body into discrete systems and treated emotional experiences as irrelevant to physical health. Dr. Sternberg's research would help to dismantle this artificial boundary, demonstrating through rigorous scientific investigation that the brain and immune system are in constant communication, their interactions mediated by hormones, neurotransmitters, and cytokines that flow between them like an ongoing conversation [1, 2].

Her work focused particularly on the body's stress response and how it affects susceptibility to disease. She discovered that the same hormonal pathways that govern our emotional responses to stress—the hypothalamic-pituitary-adrenal axis, with its cascade of cortisol and other hormones—also play a critical role in regulating inflammation and immune function [1, 4]. When stress is chronic, when the body's alarm system remains perpetually activated, the immune system becomes dysregulated. This dysregulation can manifest as increased susceptibility to infections, prolonged healing times, and the development or exacerbation of autoimmune conditions such as rheumatoid arthritis and lupus.

In 1989, Dr. Sternberg's expertise was called upon in a dramatic and unexpected way when a mysterious epidemic struck the United States. Across the country, people who had been taking L-tryptophan supplements—an amino acid sold over the counter as a treatment for insomnia, premenstrual syndrome, and depression—began developing severe muscle pain, weakness, mouth ulcers, and striking elevations in eosinophils, a type of white blood cell [1, 2]. The condition, which came to be known as eosinophilia-myalgia syndrome, ultimately affected more than 1500 people and caused at least 36 deaths [5]. Dr. Sternberg led the NIH research response and coordinated the interagency investigation that followed, working with teams from the CDC and FDA to trace the epidemic to contaminated batches of L-tryptophan manufactured by a single Japanese company using genetically modified bacteria [2].

For her outstanding contributions to understanding the L-tryptophan epidemic, Dr. Sternberg was awarded the FDA Commissioner's Special Citation in 1991 and the Public Health Service Superior Service Award in 1994 [2]. She would later reflect that she had been working in the lab as a scientist, not realizing that sometimes findings can have huge economic implications, until her work garnered such a prestigious honor. Of course, the experience reinforced the power of rigorous scientific investigation to address public health crises and protect vulnerable populations.

When asked to consider the obstacles along her path, she reflected upon the use of the word "stress," in her dialogue with fellow scientists and amongst the general public. She was initially tentative but found confidence as her scientific evidence mounted. Her research helped establish the field now known as psychoneuroimmunology: the study of how the mind, brain, and immune system interact to influence health and disease. How stress and its physiologic response was manifested in pathology. She translated this work into her first book for general audiences, "The Balance Within: The Science Connecting Health and Emotions [6]."

The book was a revelation to readers who had long suspected that their emotional lives affected their physical health but lacked the scientific framework to understand how. It provided firsthand accounts of the breakthrough experiments that revealed the physical mechanisms—the nerves, cells, and hormones—used by the brain and immune system to communicate with each other. Dr. Abraham Verghese, the celebrated physician-author, called it "a tour de force, a romp through centuries of scientific discovery written by an expert in the field [6]." Dr. Joseph Martin, Dean of Harvard Medical School, praised it as "a welcome addition at a time when considerable puzzlement and confusion exists regarding alternative or complementary medicine [6]."

"The Balance Within" answered questions that had haunted both patients and physicians: Will stress make us sick? Why do we feel sick when we get sick? How does our health affect our moods? The book explained how chronic stress leads to suppression of the immune system, stifling the body's ability to heal. It explored the placebo effect not as a curiosity to be dismissed but as evidence of the brain's remarkable capacity to influence physiological processes. And it pointed toward new therapeutic possibilities; ways of harnessing the mind-body connection to prevent illness and promote healing [6].

But Dr. Sternberg's curiosity did not stop at the internal landscape of the body. In her second major book, "Healing Spaces: The Science of Place and Well-Being" (2009) [7], she turned her attention outward, to the environments we inhabit and their effects on our health. The book was inspired in part by a personal experience of healing. During a period of professional exhaustion and physical illness, Dr. Sternberg traveled to Greece, where the experience of being immersed in beauty—the light, the architecture, the landscape—seemed to catalyze a profound restoration. She began to wonder: could there be scientific explanations for the healing power of place?

"Healing Spaces," explored this question through the lens of neuroscience and immunology. Dr. Sternberg recounted the landmark 1984 study by researcher Roger Ulrich, who found that hospital patients recovering from gallbladder surgery healed faster when their rooms had windows overlooking trees rather than brick walls [8]. The patients with nature views required less pain medication, had shorter hospital stays, and experienced fewer postoperative complications [8]. How could a pleasant view speed healing? Dr. Sternberg pursued this question through a series of places and situations—from ancient Greek healing temples to modern hospital designs, from Disney theme parks to Frank Gehry concert halls—exploring the neurobiology of the senses and how our perceptions of our environment translate into physiological responses [7].

The book demonstrated how light, sound, smell, and spatial configuration can trigger or reduce stress, induce anxiety or instill peace. It showed how the brain's stress response—the same hormonal cascade that Dr. Sternberg had studied in her laboratory research—could be activated or calmed by environmental cues. And it pointed toward practical applications: how hospitals, schools, offices, and homes could be designed to promote health and well-being rather than undermine it. The President of the American Institute of Architects recognized "Healing Spaces" as an inspiration for launching the AIA's Design and Health Initiative, reflecting the book's influence on professional practice beyond medicine [1].

In 2009, Sternberg co-created and hosted a PBS television special, *The Science of Healing with Dr. Esther Sternberg*, produced by Emmy Award-winning Resolution Pictures [9]. The program followed Sternberg to a tiny village in Greece, where her personal experience of the power of place in healing had inspired the research that became *Healing Spaces*. Viewers joined her as she explored ruins of ancient Greek healing temples and visited cutting-edge science labs to uncover the source of her healing. The program introduced a broad audience to the research revealing the many ways the brain helps us heal, both emotionally and physically [1, 9].

In 2012, after 26 years at the National Institutes of Health, Dr. Sternberg moved to the University of Arizona, where she was appointed to the Inaugural Andrew Weil Chair for Research in Integrative Medicine and became Research Director for the Andrew Weil Center for Integrative Medicine [1]. She also founded the University of Arizona Institute on Place, Wellbeing & Performance, an interdisciplinary institute that links together the expertise of the College of Medicine, the Arizona Center for Integrative Medicine, and the College of Architecture, Planning and Landscape Architecture [1–4]. In this role, she has continued to bridge the worlds of medicine, architecture, and design, translating research findings into practical applications for creating healthier environments.

The move to Arizona represented more than a change of institution; it represented an evolution in Dr. Sternberg's mission. At the University of Arizona, she found an environment uniquely suited to interdisciplinary collaboration; a place where researchers in medicine, psychology, architecture, and landscape design could work together to understand how the built and natural environments affect human health and well-being. The concept of integrative medicine, championed by Andrew Weil and central to the Center's mission, aligned perfectly with Dr. Sternberg's own vision of health as emerging from the complex interactions between mind, body, and environment [1, 3].

During the COVID-19 pandemic in the spring of 2020, Dr. Sternberg's expertise became urgently relevant as millions of people suddenly found themselves working from home, often in spaces never designed for prolonged occupancy. She presented four Public Service Announcements on AZPM addressing the challenges of this new reality: lowering stress, making your stress response work for you, making your home a healing space, and understanding the seven domains of integrative medicine [1]. Her message was that even in constrained circumstances, people could take simple steps to create environments that supported rather than undermined their well-being.

Her most recent book, "Well at Work: Creating Wellbeing in Any Workspace" (2023), brings her expertise into the post-COVID era, addressing questions that have become urgently relevant to millions of workers around the world [1, 10]. Named a Top Ten Lifestyle Book for Fall 2023 by Publishers Weekly and longlisted for the Outstanding Works of Literature Award, the book offers practical guidance on designing workspaces—whether in traditional offices or corners of bedrooms—to enhance physical and emotional well-being [1, 10, 11]. Drawing on the seven domains of integrative health—stress and resilience, movement, sleep, relationships, nutrition, spirituality, and the natural environment—Dr. Sternberg provides a menu of simple steps anyone can take to thrive wherever they work [1].

The book has received endorsements from figures as diverse as Arianna Huffington, Deepak Chopra, and the 17th Surgeon General of the United States, Richard Carmona. Rick Fedrizzi, Executive Chairman of the International WELL Building Institute, called it "a groundbreaking guide to improving employee health and well-being [1]." Gregg Easterbrook, author of "It's Better Than It Looks," observed that "Esther Sternberg consistently is 10 years ahead on psychology, spirituality and the mind-body problem. To find out what everybody will be thinking in 10 years, read 'Well at Work' today [1]."

Throughout her career, Dr. Sternberg has been recognized with numerous honors that reflect the breadth and impact of her work. She was recognized by the National Library of Medicine as one of 300 women physicians who "Changed the Face of Medicine," a distinction that acknowledges her pioneering contributions to medical science [2]. In 2012, she received the Anita B. Roberts Distinguished Women Scientists at NIH Lectureship [1]. Trinity College Dublin awarded her an honorary doctorate in medicine on the occasion of its 300th anniversary, recognizing her contributions to medical science and public health [2]. She has served as member and Chair of the National Library of Medicine's Board of Regents and has advised the World Health Organization, the U.S. National Academies of Sciences, Engineering and Medicine, the International WELL Building Institute, the Royal Society in London, and the Vatican, where she was presented to Pope Benedict XVI [1].

Her advisory role to such diverse organizations reflects the universal applicability of her research. Whether she is consulting with healthcare systems about hospital design, advising corporations about workplace wellness, or briefing government officials on public health policy, Dr. Sternberg brings the same evidence-based approach that has characterized her scientific work. She has testified before Congress, collaborated with the U.S. General Services Administration on federal building design, and worked with the U.S. Surgeon General's office on health promotion initiatives. In each of these contexts, she has served as a bridge between the world of scientific research and the world of practical application.

She has been a panelist at the United Nations, an invited delegate to Fortune Magazine's Most Powerful Women Summit, and a featured speaker at venues ranging from the Vatican's Pontifical Council for Healthcare Workers to the SXSW festival. Her work has been featured extensively in media, including CBS 60 Minutes Overtime, NPR's "On Being" with Krista Tippett, PBS, ABC News, the Washington Post, the New York Times, Forbes Magazine, and Oprah Magazine.

Dr. Sternberg's scholarly output reflects the depth and rigor of her research. She has authored over 240 scholarly articles published in leading journals including Science, Nature Reviews Immunology, Nature Medicine, The New England Journal of Medicine, Scientific American, JAMA, and Proceedings of the National Academy of Sciences. She has edited ten technical books on brain-immune connections and design and health. She writes a monthly blog for Psychology Today that has garnered tens of thousands of readers on subjects including stress and illness, gratitude and wellness, and place and well-being.

The consistency of her message across these diverse platforms—scientific journals, popular books, television programs, and public lectures—reflects a unified vision of health that transcends disciplinary boundaries. Whether she is writing for colleagues in immunology or advising architects about hospital design, Dr. Sternberg returns to the same fundamental insight: that health emerges from the complex interactions between our inner biological processes and our outer physical and social environments. This insight, once considered radical, has increasingly become part of mainstream medical thinking, thanks in large part to her work [1].

Today, Dr. Sternberg holds the title of Research Professor of Medicine (Retired) at the University of Arizona, with joint appointments in Psychology, Architecture, Planning and Landscape Architecture, and Nutritional Sciences and Wellness [1]. As Founding Director of the University of Arizona Institute on Place, Wellbeing & Performance, she continues to work with the Andrew Weil Center for Integrative Medicine and the UArizona College of Architecture, Planning & Landscape Architecture on projects related to place and well-being [1]. Most recently, she played a key role in embedding integrative health design principles in the new

Andrew Weil Center for Integrative Medicine building complex at the University of Arizona, which won Honorable Mention in The International Architecture Awards 2025. She has also founded Star Mountain LLC, a consulting firm through which she is taking her expertise in designing for well-being into the private sector [1].

She has helped to legitimize an entire field of inquiry—the science of mind-body interactions—that was once dismissed as the province of New Age healers and alternative medicine practitioners. By applying rigorous scientific methods to questions about stress, emotion, and health, she has provided physicians with evidence-based frameworks for understanding phenomena they had long observed but could not explain. Her work on the built environment and health has influenced architects, urban planners, and policymakers, contributing to a growing movement to design spaces that promote human well-being.

The implications of Dr. Sternberg's research for medical education and healthcare delivery are profound. If stress can suppress the immune system and contribute to disease, then addressing stress must become an integral part of medical treatment rather than an afterthought. These are not merely academic questions; they have direct implications for how we train physicians, design healthcare facilities, and deliver care to patients. For medical trainees struggling with burnout and seeking meaning in the concept of wellness, Dr. Sternberg's work offers scientific validation for what many have intuitively understood: that the environments in which we work profoundly affect our ability to care for ourselves and our patients. The residency workroom without windows, the hospital corridor flooded with harsh fluorescent light, the constant noise of monitors and alarms; these are not merely inconveniences but factors that actively influence our stress responses, our immune function, and our capacity for empathy and attention. Understanding this connection is the first step toward creating training environments that support rather than undermine the well-being of future physicians.

Dr. Sternberg's career demonstrates what is possible when a physician-scientist refuses to accept artificial boundaries, between mind and body, between research and practice, between the laboratory and the world. Her discoveries have given us new tools for understanding how emotions affect health, how environments shape well-being, and how the ancient intuition that believing might make you well is grounded in biological reality. In the tradition of physician-writers who use the written word to extend their influence beyond the clinic and the laboratory, Dr. Esther Sternberg has illuminated pathways that connect the most intimate experiences of our emotional lives to the most fundamental processes of our physical bodies.

References

1. Sternberg EM. Esther M. Sternberg, M.D. [Official website]. n.d. https://esthersternberg.com/.
2. National Library of Medicine. Esther M. Sternberg. Changing the Face of Medicine. n.d. https://cfmedicine.nlm.nih.gov/physicians/biography_309.html.

3. University of Arizona College of Architecture, Planning and Landscape Architecture. Esther Sternberg. n.d. https://capla.arizona.edu/faculty-staff/esther-sternberg.
4. University of Arizona College of Medicine - Tucson. Esther M Sternberg, MD. n.d. https://medicine.arizona.edu/person/esther-m-sternberg-md.
5. Allen JA, Peterson A, Sufit R, Hinchcliff ME, Mahoney JM, Wood TA, Miller FW, Whitfield ML, Varga J. Post-epidemic eosinophilia-myalgia syndrome associated with L-tryptophan. Arthritis Rheum. 2011;63(11):3633–9. https://doi.org/10.1002/art.30514.
6. Sternberg EM. The balance within: the science connecting health and emotions. Macmillan; 2001. https://www.amazon.com/Balance-Within-Science-Connecting-Emotions/dp/0716744457.
7. Sternberg EM. Healing spaces: the science of place and Well-being. Belknap Press of Harvard University Press; 2009. https://www.amazon.com/Healing-Spaces-Science-Place-Well-Being/dp/0674057481.
8. Ulrich RS. View through a window may influence recovery from surgery. Science. 1984;224(4647):420–1. https://doi.org/10.1126/science.6143402.
9. IMDb. The Science of Healing with Dr. Esther Sternberg. 2009. https://www.imdb.com/title/tt1531049/.
10. Sternberg EM. Well at work: creating wellbeing in any workspace. Little, Brown Spark; 2023. https://www.amazon.com/Well-Work-Creating-Wellbeing-Workspace-ebook/dp/B0BRKNYPX3.
11. Publishers Weekly. Well at Work: creating wellbeing in any workspace [Review]. 2023. http://www.publishersweekly.com/9780316542685.

Chapter 24
Uché Blackstock, MD

I remember my first encounter with Dr. Blackstock, on #MedTwitter in its heyday, and my initial surge of excitement at seeing my mother's Igbo name, which means Wisdom, shared by this incredible physician. She had written a letter, in exit-interview style, titled "Why Black Doctors Like Me Are Leaving Faculty Positions in Academic Medical Centers." As a resident at an academic medical center, of West African geographic ancestry, I was drawn in to the answer to a question I, myself, had pondered. I sought a career in academia; I loved teaching, I enjoyed research, I thrived in the dichotomy of inpatient and clinic care, and I was sure that my niche interest in pediatric cardio-oncology would be best supported in an academic realm. Like most trainees on a similar path, I was always seeking mentorship, the backbone of academic achievement. Finding a physician who had walked the same path you were choosing was ideal to avoid potholes and hazards on the journey. Finding one with shared demographics offered nuance in an environment guided by multiple hidden curricula. And I was lucky; although Black female physicians make up just shy of 3% of the U.S. physician workforce, one of my mentors was a Black female pediatric cardiologist in my training institution. Reading Dr. Blackstone's words, in pre-pandemic 2020, was a reminder that there remains an abundance of work to be done to meet the goal of the Department of Health and Human Services, "to achieve health equity, eliminate disparities, and improve the health of all groups." By those of us, including myself, who are within academic medicine, and by the institutions that train us.

Dr. Uché Blackstock was born on November 4, 1977, in Brooklyn, New York, into a family where medicine was not merely a profession but a calling passed down through generations [1–3]. Her mother, Dr. Dale Gloria Blackstock, had grown up in central Brooklyn, raised by a single mother on public assistance [4]. Against seemingly insurmountable odds, Dale became the first person in her family to attend college, ultimately graduating from Harvard Medical School in

O. M. Cox, *The Pen, The Stethoscope, and The Scalpel*,
https://doi.org/10.1007/978-3-032-19406-0_24

1976 and returning to her Brooklyn community as a nephrologist at Kings County Hospital Center [1, 4]. For Uché and her fraternal twin sister, Oni, their earliest memories were intertwined with the rhythms of their mother's medical practice; the smell of disinfectant in hospital hallways, the squeak of shoes on linoleum floors, the sight of their mother engaged in deep conversation with patients who were also her neighbors [1, 4].

The sisters grew up in Crown Heights, a bustling Brooklyn neighborhood that was home to middle-class and working-class families, a uniquely Brooklyn mix of Black Americans and Caribbean immigrants like their father, Earl Blackstock, who had been born in Jamaica [5–7]. Their mother was constantly reading to them as children, bringing them to the library for story time, taking them on educational adventures in Prospect Park and the Brooklyn Botanic Garden [6]. When they got older, she was the kind of mother who didn't hesitate to assign extra work if she felt their teachers weren't providing sufficient challenge [1, 7, 8]. From an early age, the Blackstock twins played with their mother's doctor's bag, an old-school, heavy black leather bag, worn and cracked around the edges, with Dale's name written in faded golden uppercase letters followed by "M.D." The bag lived under her bureau, and the girls knew it was important to her, which made it important to them [8].

Dr. Dale Blackstock was not merely a physician; she was a community health advocate decades before the term "health equity" entered the medical lexicon [8]. She served as president of an organization of Brooklyn's Black women doctors, leading a group of physicians who understood that caring for patients meant caring for the whole person, their families, their circumstances, their neighborhoods [6, 8]. When patients came to see Dr. Blackstock, they weren't merely having their blood pressure or cholesterol checked; they were meeting with someone who would assess how their whole being was faring. Growing up watching her mother practice this form of medicine, Uché assumed that most physicians were Black women like her mother, her mother's colleagues, and her own pediatrician. It would take years for her to understand how profoundly wrong that assumption was [1, 6, 8].

The twins attended Stuyvesant High School, the elite public magnet school in New York City, graduating in 1995 [6]. They then followed their mother's path to Harvard University for their undergraduate education, with Uché developing an interest in journalism and writing for The Harvard Crimson alongside her pre-medical studies. But tragedy struck during Uché's sophomore year when her mother was diagnosed with acute myelogenous leukemia. In July 1997, Dr. Dale Gloria Blackstock died at the age of 47 [8]. The twins were just 19 years old. They had lost not only their mother but their model, their inspiration, the physician whose practice had shown them what medicine could be when practiced with love, attention, and commitment to community [1, 7, 8].

Despite their grief—or perhaps because of it—both sisters continued on the path their mother had illuminated. After completing their undergraduate degrees at Harvard, Uché and Oni both enrolled at Harvard Medical School. When they graduated in 2005, they became the first Black mother-daughter legacies in the institution's history [8]. It was a distinction that spoke both to their family's remarkable achievements and to the persistent underrepresentation of Black Americans in medicine. With only about 6% of physicians in the United States being Black, and nearly 3% being Black women, the Blackstock sisters were making history simply by following in their mother's footsteps [6].

Following medical school, Dr. Uché Blackstock chose to complete her residency in emergency medicine at SUNY Downstate Medical Center in Brooklyn, the very institution affiliated with Kings County Hospital, where her mother had practiced [1, 8]. It was a deliberate choice to return to her roots, to serve the community that had shaped her. Her residency was followed by a Chief Resident year, prior to her embarking on an emergency ultrasound fellowship at Mount Sinai Morningside in 2010, developing expertise in point-of-care imaging that would later inform her academic contributions [9].

In July 2010, Dr. Blackstock was appointed as an assistant professor at the New York University School of Medicine, where she held a simultaneous position as an emergency physician [9]. Dr. Blackstock threw herself into both clinical and academic work, and in 2012, she was named Ultrasound Content Director at NYU, developing and implementing a longitudinal point-of-care ultrasound curriculum for medical students [9]. In October 2017, she was appointed Faculty Director for Recruitment, Retention and Inclusion in the Office of Diversity Affairs, where she became responsible for developing and implementing diversity, equity, and inclusion initiatives for Black, Latino, and Indigenous faculty [1, 9].

But as Dr. Blackstock would later write, her time in academic medicine revealed the profound gap between institutional rhetoric about diversity and the lived reality of Black faculty members. She found herself expected to execute "diversity" efforts—chairing diversity committees, mentoring minority trainees—while rarely being recognized or compensated for this invaluable work [1, 10]. She experienced what she described as a toxic work environment that included sexism, racism, and denial of promotion [10]. The irony was not lost on her: Black faculty members were being tasked with remedying the outcomes of centuries of institutional racism that they had not created in the first place. The work was exhausting, isolating, and ultimately unsustainable [1, 8, 10].

In 2019, Dr. Blackstock made a decision that would alter the trajectory of her career. She left NYU School of Medicine and founded Advancing Health Equity, an organization dedicated to partnering with healthcare institutions to dismantle racism in healthcare and close the gap in racial health inequities [10]. It was a leap of faith—leaving the security of academic medicine for the uncertainty of entrepreneurship—but it was also a recognition that the change she wanted to create could not happen from within institutions resistant to transformation [1, 11]. Through Advancing Health Equity, Dr. Blackstock began facilitating trainings with healthcare organizations on unconscious bias, structural racism, and health equity, while also providing consulting services to support organizations in achieving their health equity goals [11]. Clients have included major companies, hospitals, and health systems seeking to create strategic plans for promoting equitable healthcare [11].

In January 2020, just weeks before the COVID-19 pandemic would transform American life, Dr. Blackstock published the op-ed in STAT News titled "Why Black Doctors Like Me Are Leaving Faculty Positions in Academic Medical Centers [10]." The piece was a call to arms, articulating what many Black physicians had experienced but few had stated so publicly. She noted that a decade earlier, the Department of Health and Human Services had made achieving health equity one of its goals for Healthy People 2020, and that the nation had not come close [10]. Black Americans continued to experience some of the worst health outcomes of any racial group: Black men had the shortest life expectancies, Black women had the highest maternal mortality rates, Black babies had the highest infant mortality rates [10]. Diversifying the healthcare workforce was one solution, but that was a tall order when healthcare work environments remained unwelcoming and discriminatory to Black healthcare providers.

The piece resonated deeply with Black physicians across the country. Many reached out to Dr. Blackstock to share their own experiences of isolation, discrimination, and burnout in academic medicine. Her words gave voice to a collective frustration that had long simmered beneath the surface of professional decorum. As she would later reflect, "I wasn't just writing it for myself. I knew it wasn't just my experience, even though at the time, I felt very alone [8, 10]."

Then came the pandemic. As COVID-19 swept through the United States in early 2020, Dr. Blackstock was working part-time at several urgent care centers in Brooklyn, treating patients who presented with the symptoms of coronavirus disease [9]. She noticed something troubling: the patients were "getting browner and browner by the day [12]." The pandemic was exposing and amplifying the racial health inequities that Dr. Blackstock had spent her career studying. Black and Latino communities were being devastated by the virus at rates far exceeding their white counterparts, a disparity rooted in the same structural racism that produced inequities in housing, employment, environmental exposure, and access to healthcare [1, 9, 11].

Dr. Blackstock became a vital voice during the pandemic, using her expertise and her platform to explain these disparities to the public [1]. She spoke and wrote about the potential racial health inequities that would be exposed and amplified by the pandemic, and what federal, state, and local officials needed to do to mitigate the virus spread among the country's most vulnerable populations [1, 13]. Throughout the crisis, she appeared consistently on podcasts, radio, digital media, and network news, committed to conveying responsible and accurate information about COVID-19. In June 2020, Yahoo! News invited her to become a Medical Contributor for the network, a role that expanded her reach even further [1, 14].

Her media presence and accolades continued to grow. Dr. Blackstock became a regular contributor on MSNBC and NBC News, where her expert analysis of health equity issues reached millions of viewers. Her writing appeared in The Chicago Tribune, Scientific American, The Washington Post, and STAT News [1]. She was featured on CNN, NPR's Morning Edition, The Brian Lehrer Show, PBS NewsHour, and in Essence magazine. She spoke at panels at Afropunk and Essence Fest, bringing her message to diverse audiences beyond traditional medical and media circles. Forbes described her as "a growing voice that is bringing to light and offering solutions to unconscious bias and structural racism among healthcare organizations [15]." In 2021, Dr. Blackstock received the American Medical Women's Association Presidential Award [16] and was named Harvard Humanist of the Year [17]. And in 2024, TIME magazine included her among its "100 Most Influential People in Global Health," a testament to how far her voice had traveled from that STAT News op-ed 4 years earlier [18].

But it would be the written word that would become Dr. Blackstock's most enduring contribution. In the summer of 2020, she received an unexpected email from a literary agent who had been following her work. "I think you have a story to tell," the agent wrote, "and you're the only person to tell that story [19]." Dr. Blackstock had never considered writing a book, but the invitation sparked something. The story she had to tell was one of growing up as the daughter of a Black woman physician who was doing health equity work before there was a name for it. It was the story of a first-year medical student whose appendicitis was misdiagnosed multiple times—perhaps because she was a young Black woman—leading to a ruptured appendix, complications, and missed classes. It was the story of a physician who had to unlearn what she had been taught and recognize the gaps in her education and training [8].

"Legacy: A Black Physician Reckons with Racism in Medicine," was published by Viking Books on January 23, 2024 [8, 20]. It became an instant New York Times bestseller. The book is at once a searing indictment of the American healthcare system, a generational family memoir, and a call to action. It traces Dr. Blackstock's odyssey from child to medical student to practicing physician, to finally seizing her own power as a health equity advocate against the backdrop of the pandemic. But at its heart, the book is a love letter to her mother, the original Dr. Blackstock, whose life was devoted to serving her community and who died too young, possibly as a result of environmental exposures in the very Brooklyn neighborhoods she served. Dr. Uché Blackstock notes in the book that there are two radioactive dumping grounds in Black and Latinx communities in Brooklyn, where her mother lived [8, 20].

The reviews were powerful. Dr. Abraham Verghese, the celebrated physician-author, called the book "both a compelling memoir and an edifying analysis of the inequities in the way we deliver healthcare in America. Uché Blackstock is a force of nature [20]." Jacqueline Woodson, the National Book Award-winning author, wrote that after reading "Legacy," so many of us will find "…that we are ready for the fight [20]." Gayle King, on CBS Mornings, declared that the book "should be required reading for all medical students [20]."

Today, Dr. Uché Blackstock continues her work at the intersection of medicine, advocacy, and public communication. She still practices clinically, working part-time at urgent care centers in Brooklyn, maintaining the patient contact that keeps her grounded in the realities of healthcare delivery. Through Advancing Health Equity, which celebrated its fifth anniversary in 2024, she continues to help major companies, hospitals, and health systems create strategic plans for promoting equitable healthcare. And her research and advocacy have informed policy decisions at local, state, and national levels [1].

Her work with Advancing Health Equity reflects a practical approach to systemic change. Rather than merely diagnosing the problems within healthcare institutions, Dr. Blackstock works with organizations to develop concrete solutions [1, 11]. She conducts trainings on unconscious bias and structural racism, helps organizations develop diversity and inclusion strategies, and consults on creating work environments where clinicians of all backgrounds can thrive. The organization has partnered with major healthcare systems, pharmaceutical companies, and nonprofits, translating academic insights about health equity into actionable institutional change [11]. For Dr. Blackstock, this work represents the logical extension of her clinical practice; healing not just individual patients but the systems that shape their care.

In her public speaking, Blackstock often asks audiences to consider a question: What is your legacy going to be? It is a question she asks herself, reflecting on the path her mother laid and the path she is now forging. Her mother wrote, 30 years ago, that "it is ironic that as we enter the age of neotechnology, we do not have a health-care system in place that is equitable for all participants. Worse, a health-care system that refuses to embrace all in need [8, 20]." Those words remain devastatingly relevant today. The statistics that Dr. Blackstock cites in her writing and speaking—that Black babies are more than twice as likely as white babies to die in their first year of life, that the richest Black mothers and their babies are twice as likely to die as the richest white mothers and their babies—reflect systemic failures that transcend individual behavior or choice.

The publication of "Legacy" positioned Dr. Blackstock as a leading voice in what might be called the health equity literary movement; a growing body of work that uses narrative to illuminate systemic injustice in healthcare. Her book has been adopted as required reading in medical schools and nursing programs, used in diversity campus read programs at institutions like UMass Chan Medical School, and discussed at professional conferences across the country [21]. Her work has highlighted the role of the Flexner Report in shaping the landscape of medical education and its role in perpetuating racial exclusion [22]. She has advocated for curricula that address the historical and ongoing impact of racism on health outcomes, moving beyond the superficial inclusion of "diversity" content to a fundamental reconsideration of how medicine is taught and practiced.

"Although she died prematurely," Dr. Blackstock writes in "Legacy," "my mother's spirit lives on in my sister and me, her patients, the communities she served, the future physicians she mentored, and the organizations she led. It will live on in this book too." And indeed it does. In the tradition of physician-writers who use their pens to extend their healing influence beyond the clinic, Dr. Uché Blackstock has written herself into the ongoing story of American medicine, and in doing so, has honored the legacy of the remarkable woman who first showed her what a physician could be.

References

1. Blackstock U. Dr. Uché Blackstock [Official website]. n.d. https://ucheblackstock.com/.
2. Harvard Medicine Magazine. Uché Blackstock is on a mission to root out racism in medicine. 2024. https://magazine.hms.harvard.edu/articles/uche-blackstock-mission-root-out-racism-medicine.
3. Penguin Random House. Uché Blackstock, MD. n.d. https://www.penguinrandomhouse.com/authors/2265713/uche-blackstock-md/.
4. Essence. Black moms on the front lines: twin doctors Uché and Oni Blackstock are battling structural racism in medicine for Black lives. 2020, May 22. https://www.essence.com/feature/black-moms-front-lines-twin-doctors-uche-oni-blackstock-battling-structural-racism-in-medicine/.
5. Gorce TL. How Oni and Uché Blackstock, doctors, spend their Sundays. The New York Times. 2022, March 18. https://www.nytimes.com/2022/03/18/nyregion/oni-and-uche-blackstock.html.
6. Offenback L. How Dr. Uché Blackstock is prescribing equity for America's healthcare system. MM+M—Medical Marketing and Media. 2025, August 28. https://www.mmm-online.com/news/how-dr-uche-blackstock-is-prescribing-equity-for-americas-healthcare-system/.
7. Cohen J. After a life together, living apart. The New York Times. 2006, February 12. https://www.nytimes.com/2006/02/12/realestate/after-a-life-together-living-apart.html.
8. Blackstock U. Legacy: a black physician reckons with racism in medicine. Viking Books; 2024. https://www.penguinrandomhouse.com/books/705871/legacy-by-uche-blackstock-md/.
9. EMRA. Emergency medicine 45 under 45: Dr. Blackstock. 2019. https://www.emra.org/be-involved/awards/45under45/2019/uche-blackstock-45.
10. Blackstock U. Why Black doctors like me are leaving faculty positions in academic medical centers. STAT News. 2020, January 16. https://www.statnews.com/2020/01/16/black-doctors-leaving-faculty-positions-academic-medical-centers/.
11. Advancing Health Equity. About. n.d. https://advancinghealthequity.com/about/.
12. Falci M. Dr Uché Blackstock speaks on racism in medicine. Clinical Advisor. 2025, February 4. https://www.clinicaladvisor.com/features/dr-uche-blackstock-speaks-on-racism-in-medicine/.
13. Blackstock U. [@uche_blackstock]. Tweets [X profile]. X. n.d. https://x.com/uche_blackstock.
14. Yahoo Finance. Yahoo News medical contributor on life post COVID-19 vaccine: "We probably will be living with the virus for a while even after a vaccine." [Video]. 2020, September 21. https://finance.yahoo.com/video/yahoo-news-medical-contributor-life-201429671.html.
15. Reid M. Why going to the doctor as a Black person is hard. Forbes. 2020, February 11 https://www.forbes.com/sites/maryannreid/2020/02/10/why-going-to-the-doctor-as-a-black-person-is-hard/.
16. American Medical Women's Association. American Medical Women's Association 2021 awards. 2021. http://amwa-doc.org/wp-content/uploads/2025/11/AMWA-2021-Awards-Info-Public-2-11.pdf.

17. Humanist Chaplaincy at Harvard. Harvard humanist of the year for 2021 is Dr. Uché Blackstock. 2021, November 2. https://www.humanistchaplaincy.org/post/humanist-of-the-year-2021.
18. Ducharme J. Uché Blackstock. TIME. 2024, May 2. https://time.com/6967230/dr-uche-blackstock/.
19. Mooney S. A conversation with Dr. Uché Blackstock. MedCentral. 2025, January 17 https://www.medcentral.com/biz-policy/legacy-author-physician-uche-blackstock-racism-in-medicine.
20. Blackstock U. Legacy: a black physician reckons with racism in medicine. Viking; 2024. https://www.amazon.com/Legacy-Physician-Reckons-Racism-Medicine/dp/0593491289.
21. Innis J. UMass Chan launches 2024 diversity campus read with legacy: a Black physician reckons with racism in medicine. UMass Chan Medical School. 2024, January 30. https://www.umassmed.edu/news/news-archives/2024/01/umass-chan-launches-2024-diversity-campus-read-with-legacy-a-black-physician-reckons-with-racism/.
22. Mosley T. Following in her mom's footsteps, a doctor fights to make medicine more inclusive. NPR. 2024, January 22. https://www.npr.org/2024/01/22/1226047324/uche-blackstock-legacy-racism-medicine.

Index

O. M. Cox, *The Pen, The Stethoscope, and The Scalpel*,
https://doi.org/10.1007/978-3-032-19406-0

GPSR Compliance

The European Union's (EU) General Product Safety Regulation (GPSR) is a set of rules that requires consumer products to be safe and our obligations to ensure this.

If you have any concerns about our products, you can contact us on ProductSafety@springernature.com

In case Publisher is established outside the EU, the EU authorized representative is:

Springer Nature Customer Service Center GmbH
Europaplatz 3
69115 Heidelberg, Germany

Batch number: 10370708

Printed by Printforce, the Netherlands